Heloise Gadd .

Austral

FIRST AID

Australian
FIRST AID

AN AUTHORISED MANUAL OF
ST JOHN AMBULANCE
AUSTRALIA

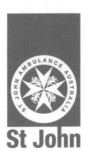

St John Ambulance Australia
Canberra Avenue
Forrest ACT 2603

© St John Ambulance Australia 1998
First edition 1984
Reprinted with corrections 1984-1988
Second edition completely rewritten 1989
Reprinted with corrections 1990-1998
Third edition completely rewritten 1998
Reprinted with corrections 7/1999, 11/1999, 6/2000,
1/2001, 10/2001

ISBN 0 949569 38 0

Editors: Vic Groenhout, Glen Rogers, Peter Bowler,
Shirley Dyson
Designer: Derrick I. Stone, Goro Jankulovski
Photographer: Chris Groenhout
Illustrator: Dr Levent Efe
Production management: Acute Image Pty Ltd
Copyedit: Perfect Words

Typeset in Palatino
Colour separation and reproduction by
Impact Printing (Melbourne)
Printed and bound by
Impact Printing (Melbourne)

FOREWORD

It is a wonderful thing to save a life. It is also wonderful to know that we have the simple skills to preserve life if, at any moment, we are confronted with an emergency. First aid training empowers us to do the best for those who, usually unexpectedly and often through no fault of their own, suddenly need our care.

Every member of the community, at some time, need to administer first aid. Every parent will. Every workmate will. Every motorist will need to give help, or have the option to give emergency aid, at some time during their driving life. Every partner will need to offer help during acute illness or injury. If that help is skilled and follows the principles taught in this book, convalescence will always be smoother and often shorter, and in many cases life itself can be preserved. In more than half the cases in which you give first aid in the future, it will be to your child or partner, or to a friend or workmate.

This book will teach you about your body—how it is made, how it functions, and how to take care of your own injuries. In this sense no other manual is more important. Most who learn the principles and practice of first aid enjoy the task, and many find it enormously enjoyable and fulfilling. The details of this text are the result of extensive experience, the distilled wisdom of a hundred years of expertise, and of the most up-to-date research.

Enjoy this book—an Australian bestseller—and become one of the million Australians who, like you, have joined the ranks of trained first aiders.

Professor John Pearn
Director of Training
St John Ambulance Australia

Contents

This is a guide to the basic first aid procedures needed in an emergency. It outlines essentials in convenient ready-reference form. Refer to the full text of later chapters for more comprehensive explanations. Remember, first aid skills are best acquired by completing a course with a Registered Training Organisation such as St John Ambulance Australia.

The St John DRABC Action Plan is a vital aid to the first aider in assessing whether the casualty has any life-threatening conditions and if any immediate first aid is necessary.

DRABC

D check for **DANGER**
- ▶ to you
- ▶ to others
- ▶ to casualty

R check **RESPONSE**
- ▶ is casualty conscious?
- ▶ is casualty unconscious?

A check **AIRWAY**
- ▶ is airway clear of objects?
- ▶ is airway open?

B check for **BREATHING**
- ▶ is chest rising and falling?
- ▶ can you hear casualty's breathing?
- ▶ can you feel the breath on your cheek?

C check for **CIRCULATION**
- ▶ can you feel a pulse?
- ▶ can you see any obvious signs of life?

E

Emergency first aid a quick guide

HANDLING AN EMERGENCY

1 ASSESS THE SCENE

Is there a danger to yourself, casualty or others?

IF NO GO TO STEP 2

IF YES THEN

If possible, remove danger— but do not put yourself at risk,

or

if possible, remove casualty from danger.

GO TO STEP 2

2 ASSESS CASUALTY

Is casualty conscious?

Shake and shout for response.

IF YES GO TO STEP 3

IF NO THEN

If others present, send them to call an ambulance ☎ **CALL 000.**

Place casualty in recovery position.

Is condition due to injury, drowning, or is casualty a child?

IF YES THEN

Go to Step 4, then resuscitate for 1 minute.

Then, if casualty still not breathing and if you are alone, call an ambulance ☎ **CALL 000.**

IF NO THEN

Assume heart failure.

Clear and open airway.

Check for breathing—up to 10 seconds.

If not breathing call an ambulance ☎ **CALL 000.** On return, go to Step 4 then commence resuscitation.

3 MONITOR VITAL SIGNS

level of consciousness

breathing

pulse

skin colour

Head-to-toe examination

MANAGE wounds and bleeding shock

Call for an ambulance if necessary ☎ **CALL 000.**

4
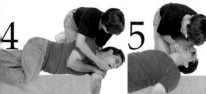

CLEAR AIRWAY & CHECK BREATHING

Clear and open airway—remove any foreign objects.

Tilt head back and slightly down and support jaw.

Check for breathing—up to 10 seconds.

Is casualty breathing?

IF **NO** GO TO STEP **5**

IF **YES** THEN

Place casualty in recovery position and carry out head-to-toe examination.

MANAGE

wounds and bleeding

shock.

5
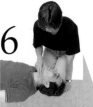

PERFORM EAR

Turn casualty onto back.

ADULT
Give two effective breaths.

INFANT/CHILD
Give two effective puffs or light breaths.

Ensure chest rise with each breath.

Has breathing returned?

IF **NO** GO TO STEP **6**

IF **YES** THEN

Place casualty in recovery position and carry out head-to-toe examination.

MANAGE

wounds and bleeding

shock.

6

CHECK FOR CIRCULATION

ADULT/CHILD
Feel for carotid pulse —up to 10 seconds.

INFANT
Feel for brachial pulse—up to 10 seconds.

Check for any movement, including swallowing.

Is pulse present?

IF **NO** GO TO STEP **7**

IF **YES** THEN

Continue EAR and check pulse about every minute until breathing resumes.

ADULT
Breathe at the rate of 15 breaths per minute.

INFANT/CHILD
Breathe at the rate of 20 breaths per minute.

7
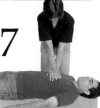

PERFORM CPR

ADULT
Alternate 15 compressions with 2 breaths at 4 cycles per minute.

INFANT/CHILD
Alternate 5 compressions with 1 breath at 12 cycles per minute.

Check pulse about every minute.

STOP CPR IF:
casualty shows signs of life

qualified help arrives

you are physically unable to continue.

If breathing resumes place casualty in recovery position.
Manage
wounds, bleeding, shock.

RECOVERY POSITION

ADULT/CHILD (from age 1)

1 **Position casualty's legs:**
  - kneel beside casualty
  - straighten casualty's limbs
  - lift nearer leg at knee so it is fully bent upwards.

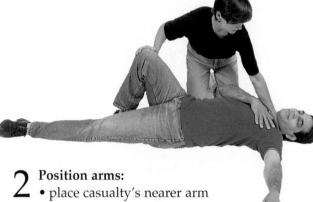

2 **Position arms:**
  - place casualty's nearer arm across chest
  - place farther arm at right angles to body.

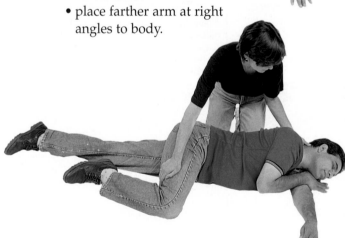

3 Roll casualty into position:
- roll casualty away from you onto side
- keep leg at right angles, with knee touching ground to prevent casualty rolling onto face.

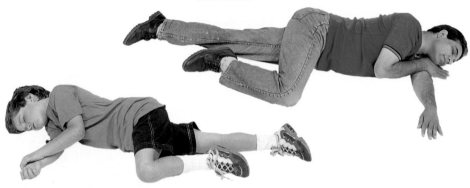

Recovery position for a child

4 Make casualty steady:
- make any adjustments necessary to ensure casualty does not roll.

5 Ensure airway is open.

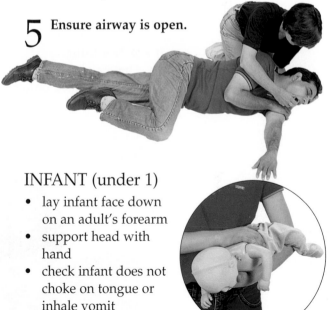

INFANT (under 1)

- lay infant face down on an adult's forearm
- support head with hand
- check infant does not choke on tongue or inhale vomit

Expired Air Resuscitation (EAR)

ADULT

1 **Clear airway:**
  - place casualty in recovery position
  - lift chin and open mouth
  - use finger to remove any obvious obstruction
  - tilt head back gently
  - check breathing for up to 10 seconds.

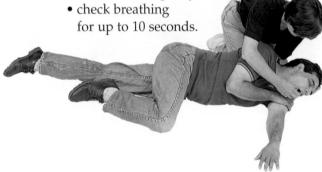

If not breathing:

2 **Open airway:**
  - turn casualty onto back
  - gently tilt head back
  - pinch nose closed (use thumb and index finger)
  - open mouth and maintain chin lift.

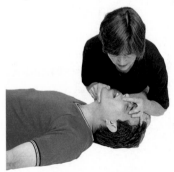

3 Give EAR (mouth-to-mouth resuscitation):

- take a full breath and place lips on casualty's mouth (ensure good seal)
- blow steadily into mouth for 1.5–2 seconds
- watch for chest to rise
- take mouth away and watch for chest to fall
- take another breath and repeat sequence, to give two effective breaths.

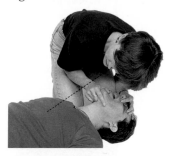

4 Check for pulse:

- check pulse at neck or wrist
- if pulse absent, commence CPR *(see p. E 10)*
- if pulse present, continue EAR at 15 breaths per minute
- recheck pulse and look for other signs of recovery about every minute.

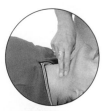 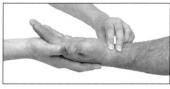

5 Place in recovery position when breathing returns.

EXPIRED AIR RESUSCITATION (EAR)

INFANT (under 1 year)
CHILD (aged 1–8)

1 **Clear airway:**
- place infant/child in recovery position
- lift chin and open mouth
- use finger to remove any obvious obstruction

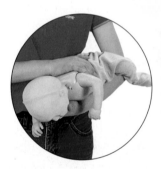

Infant recovery position

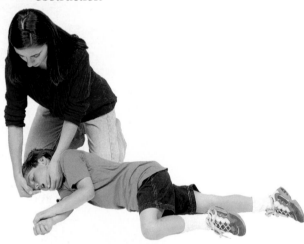

- tilt head back very gently
- check breathing for up to 10 seconds.

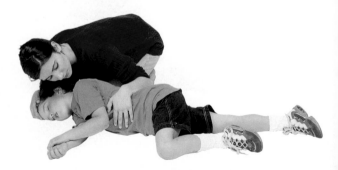

If not breathing:

2 Open airway:

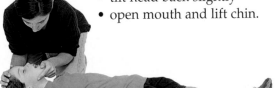

- turn casualty onto back
- tilt head back slightly
- open mouth and lift chin.

3 Give EAR (mouth-to-mouth resuscitation):
- cover mouth and nose with your mouth
- give two gentle breaths/puffs into child's/infant's mouth and nose
- check pulse—infant on inside upper arm, child at neck or wrist

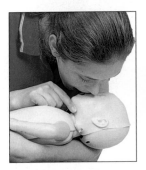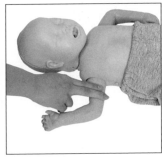

- if pulse absent, commence CPR *(see p. E-12)*
- if pulse present, continue EAR at 20 breaths per minute
- recheck pulse and look for other signs of recovery about every minute.

4 Place in recovery position when breathing returns.

NOTE

CPR combines chest compressions
with expired air resuscitation (EAR).

CPR is given when casualty is not breathing and has no pulse.

CARDIOPULMONARY RESUSCITATION (CPR)

ADULT

1 **Position hands for CPR:**
 * place casualty on back
 * find groove at neck between collarbones
 * find lower end of breastbone by running finger along last rib to centre of body
 * extend thumbs equal distances to meet in middle of breastbone

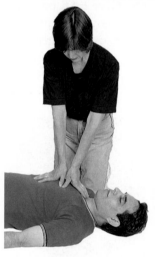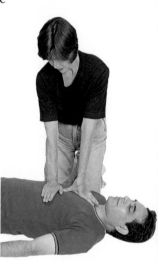

 * keep thumb of one hand in position and place heel of other hand below it
 * place heel of other hand on top of first and interlock fingers of both hands.

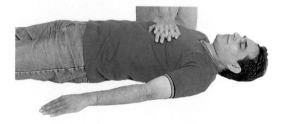

2 Commence chest compressions:

- position yourself vertically above casualty's chest
- with your arms straight, press down on breastbone to depress it about 4–5 cms
- release pressure.

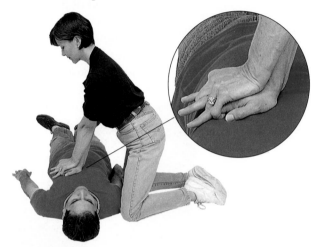

3 Continue CPR:

- complete 15 compressions
- give two effective breaths (EAR)
- continue compressions and breaths in ratio of 15:2 at a rate of 4 cycles per minute
- check pulse about every minute.

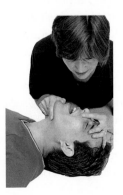
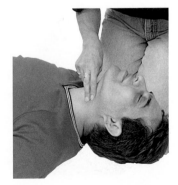

CARDIOPULMONARY RESUSCITATION (CPR)

CHILD (aged 1–8)

- use heel of one hand over lower half of breastbone to give chest compressions
- compress chest approximately 1/3 depth of chest
- give 5 chest compressions in 3 seconds
- give 1 effective breath (EAR)
  - continue compressions and breaths in ratio of 5:1 at a rate of 12 cycles per minute
    - check pulse about every minute

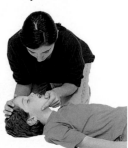
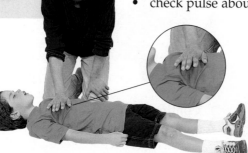

INFANT (under 1 year)

- place tips of 2 fingers (index and middle) on lower half of breastbone
- compress chest approximately 1/3 depth of chest
- give 5 chest compressions in 3 seconds
- give 1 effective breath
- continue compressions and breaths in ratio of 5:1 at a rate of 12 cycles per minute
- check pulse about every minute

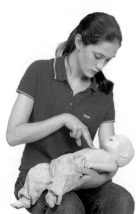

SHOCK

SIGNS & SYMPTOMS

- weak, rapid pulse
- cold, clammy skin
- rapid breathing
- faintness/dizziness
- nausea
- pale face, finger-nails, lips

1 **Lie casualty down:**
- protect casualty from cold ground
- calm casualty.

2 **Assess casualty:**
- follow DRABC.

3 ☎ *Call 000 for an ambulance.*

4 **Manage any injuries:**
- control any bleeding
- raise legs (unless fractured) above heart level
- dress any wounds or burns
- immobilise fractures.

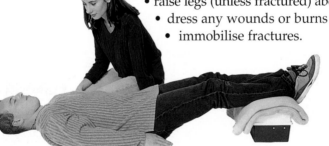

5 **Ensure comfort:**
- loosen any tight clothing around neck, chest or waist
- maintain body warmth (do not heat)
- if thirsty, moisten lips (but nothing to drink or eat).

6 **Monitor breathing and pulse:**
- maintain a clear and open airway.

7 **Place casualty in recovery position:**
- place in recovery position if casualty has difficulty breathing, is likely to vomit or becomes unconscious.

CHOKING

ADULT

Partial blockage:

- encourage casualty to relax and breathe deeply
- ask casualty to cough
- if unsuccessful, bend casualty well forward and give 4 sharp blows between shoulder-blades

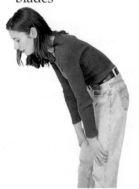
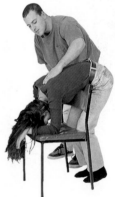

- if still unsuccessful, place casualty on side on floor ☎ *call 000 for an ambulance*

Total blockage:

- lie casualty on side on floor
- give 4 sharp blows between shoulderblades
- if unsuccessful, give 4 quick downward lateral chest thrusts (place your hands on side of chest, below casualty's armpit)
- if still unsuccessful
  ☎ *call 000 for an ambulance*
- repeat steps until help arrives or blockage clears
- follow DRABC

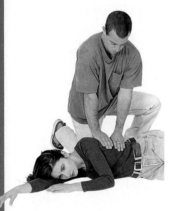

DRABC ▶

CHOKING

NOTE

Older child (from age 9)
—manage as for adult.

CHILD (1–8 years)
Partial blockage:
- ask child to try to cough up obstruction
- if unsuccessful, place child with head low and face down
- give 4 sharp blows between the shoulder-blades

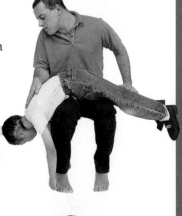

Total blockage:
- place child face down on the floor or across your lap
- give 4 sharp blows between shoulderblades
- if not breathing, give up to 4 quick, squeezing lateral chest thrusts on both sides simultaneously (place your hands below child's armpits)
- if still unsuccessful ☎ *call 000 for an ambulance*
- repeat above steps until help arrives or blockage clears
- if not breathing, follow DRABC

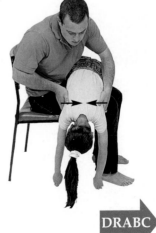

DRABC

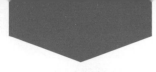

CHOKING

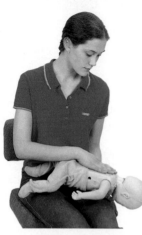

INFANT (to 1 year)

Partial blockage:
- lie infant face down on your forearm with head low
- support infant's head and shoulders on your hand
- give 4 sharp slaps between shoulders
- check in infant's mouth and remove any obstruction that has come loose
- if unsuccessful
  - ☎ *call 000 for an ambulance*

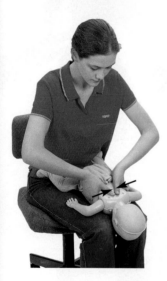

Total blockage:
- place infant face down on your lap
- give 4 sharp slaps between shoulders and check for signs of breathing
- if not breathing, give 4 quick squeezing lateral chest thrusts on both sides simultaneously (place your hands below infant's armpits)
- check in infant's mouth and remove any obstruction that has come loose
- if still unsuccessful
  - ☎ *call 000 for an ambulance*
- repeat above steps until help arrives or blockage clears
- follow DRABC

CHEST PAIN OR DISCOMFORT

Angina

- pain or discomfort in centre of chest

- pain radiating to neck and arms

- onset with exercise or emotional stress

- pain relieved by rest or medication

Heart attack

signs and symptoms similar to angina, and may include:

- severe, vice-like chest pain

- anxiety/confusion

- shortness of breath

- nausea/vomiting

- irregular pulse

- sometimes immediate collapse

WARNING: Treat situation as life-threatening.

1 **Advise casualty to rest:**
- advise casualty to stop any activity, and sit or lie down and rest.

2 **Casualty to take medication:**
- if casualty has medication for angina, get it and assist casualty in taking it.

3 **Seek urgent medical attention:**
- if unconscious, follow DRABC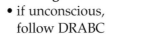
  ☎ *call 000 for an ambulance immediately*
- do not drive casualty to hospital, in case of cardiac arrest.

4 **Give aspirin:**
- give 300 mg (one tablet) of aspirin in water
- do not give aspirin to those allergic to it, to asthmatics or those on anti-coagulant medication (e.g. warfarin).

5 **Monitor vital signs:**
- monitor pulse, breathing, consciousness, skin colour
- be prepared to give CPR *(see E 10).*

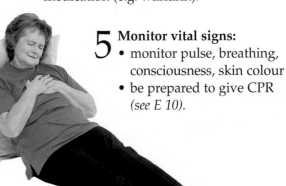

Use of Oxygen in First Aid

Detailed information on oxygen administration is found in Chapter 20—Advanced Resuscitation.

Casualties suffering from a lack of oxygen due to an injury (e.g. head injury) or medical condition (e.g. heart attack, asthma attack, shock, capsicum spray exposure, gas or smoke inhalation etc.) which may result in unconsciousness, will benefit if given oxygen. Administer oxygen if available and you have been trained to do so.

For a breathing casualty, turn oxygen on and set aflow rate of 8 lpm. Connect the oxygen delivery tube to the oxygen nipple on the mask. Place mask on casualty and instruct them to breathe normally. Remove non-return valve if present for easier exhalation.

During resuscitation of a non-breathing casualty, use oxygen at a flow rate of 15 lpm, connecting the oxygen delivery tube to the oxygen nipple on the resuscitation mask while performing mouth to mask resuscitation—this will increase the amount of oxygen the casualty is receiving.

☎ *Call 000 for an ambulance.*

DEFIBRILLATION

In a casualty suffering a sudden cardiac arrest, the electrical signals that cause the heartbeat to become chaotic and the heart stops pumping blood. The electrical shock given by a defibrillator stops this chaotic electrical activity and often then allows the heart to start beating again.

WARNING

Do not use a defibrillator:

- on a person under 12 years old

- in a moving vehicle

Before defibrillation—move:
- casualty if touching metal fixture or lying in water

- oxygen away from casualty

- mobile phones/two-way radios 2 metres away

A semi-automatic external defibrillator can be safely used on a casualty with cardiac arrest. However, good CPR is still essential before defibrillation to improve the likely outcome for the casualty. Defibrillation is most effective when carried out within three minutes of a cardiac arrest.

- follow DRABC
- if casualty is unconscious, not breathing and has no pulse, call for help and ask someone to get the defibrillator
- commence CPR and continue until defibrillator arrives
- expose the casualty's chest and follow the voice prompts
- attach adhesive pads as shown

Ask everyone to stand clear, do not touch the casualty while defibrillator is analysing—follow the voice prompts.

If the machine indicates to press the shock button—make sure everyone is clear.

If the heart re-starts, the casualty may start to regain some colour and you may be able to feel a pulse—they may start to breathe.

Monitor pulse and breathing. Continue to assist with casualty's breathing—add oxygen if available and continue until help arrives.

NOTE

Where permitted under local legislation/ regulations and if necessary:

Use another person's reliever inhaler or use one from a first aid kit to assist a casualty with a severe asthma attack.

If someone is exhibiting difficulty breathing, but has not previously had an asthma attack, assist in giving 4 puffs of a reliever and continue with 4 puffs every 4 minutes if required until an ambulance arrives.

ASTHMA ATTACK

If casualty unconscious:
- follow DRABC
- ☎ *call 000 for an ambulance*

If casualty conscious:

1 **Make casualty comfortable:**
- help casualty into comfortable position— usually sitting upright and leaning foward
- ensure adequate fresh air
- tell casualty to take slow, deep breaths.

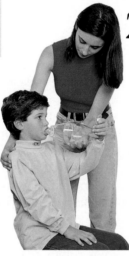

2 **Help with administration of casualty's medication:**
- give 4 puffs of a blue reliever inhaler—casualty takes a breath with each puff
- use a spacer if available: give 4 puffs, one at a time—casualty takes 4 breaths after each puff
- wait 4 minutes
- if no improvement, give another 4 puffs.

3 **If attack continues:**
- ☎ *call 000 for an ambulance*
- for a severe attack, until ambulance arrives, keep giving:
  children 4 puffs every 4 minutes
  adults   6–8 puffs every 5 minutes.

SEVERE BLEEDING

1 **Apply pressure to the wound:**
- remove or cut casualty's clothing to expose wound
- apply direct pressure over wound
- cover wound with sterile dressing
- apply a pad.

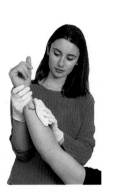

2 **Raise and support injured part:**
- lie casualty down
- raise injured part above level of heart
- handle gently if you suspect a fracture.

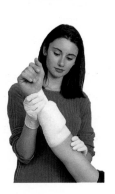

3 **Bandage wound:**
- bandage firmly in place
- apply another dressing or pad if bleeding continues.

4 **Check circulation below wound.**

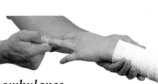

5 ☎ *Call 000 for an ambulance if severe bleeding persists.*

6 **Treat for shock:**
- see 'Shock' *(E 13)*.

BURNS

1 **Remove casualty from danger:**
- follow DRABC
- if clothing on fire:
  STOP, DROP AND ROLL
  - pull casualty to ground
  - wrap in blanket or similar
  - roll casualty along ground until flames extinguished.

DRABC

2 **Cool the burnt area:**
- hold burnt area under cold running water—at least 10 minutes
- if a chemical burn, run cold water over burnt area—at least 20 minutes
- if a bitumen burn, run cold water over burnt area for 30 minutes
- if burn is to eye, flush eye with water for 20 minutes.

3 **Remove any constrictions:**
- remove clothing and jewellery from burnt area (unless sticking to the burn).

4 **Cover burn:**
- place sterile, non-stick dressing over burn.

5 **Calm casualty.**

6 ☎ *Call 000 for an ambulance.*

SNAKE AND SPIDER BITE

SIGNS & SYMPTOMS

Snakebite
- puncture marks
- nausea, vomiting, diarrhoea
- headache
- double or blurred vision
- breathing difficulties
- drowsiness, giddiness
- pain or tightness in chest or abdomen
- respiratory weakness or arrest

Spider bite
- sharp pain
- profuse sweating
- nausea, vomiting, diarrhoea

Funnel-web spider
- copious saliva
- confusion leading to unconsciousness
- muscular twitching
- breathing difficulty

Red-back spider
- intense pain, spreading
- small hairs stand on end

WARNING

Do not wash venom off the skin as retained venom will assist identification.

Do not cut bitten area or try to suck venom out of wound.

Do not use a constrictive bandage (i.e. arterial tourniquet).

Do not try to catch the snake.

SNAKE/FUNNEL-WEB SPIDER

1 **Check breathing and pulse:**
- if casualty unconscious, follow DRABC.

2 **Calm casualty.**

3 **Apply pressure immobilisation bandage:**
- apply a firm roller bandage starting just above the fingers or toes and moving up the limb as far as can be reached
- bandage needs to be firm, as for a sprain, but not too tight.

4 **Immobilise casualty:**
- apply a splint to immobilise bitten limb
- check circulation in fingers or toes
- if possible, ensure casualty does not move.

5 ☎ *Call 000 for an ambulance.*

RED-BACK SPIDER

1 **Apply icepack to bitten area and seek medical aid.**

POISONING

- abdominal pain

- drowsiness

- nausea/vomiting

- burning pains from mouth to stomach

- difficulty in breathing

- tight chest

- blurred vision

- odours on breath

- change of skin colour with blueness around lips

- sudden collapse

WARNING

Do not attempt to induce vomiting unless advised to by Poisons Information Centre.

Cyanide Poisoning—if breathing stops, wash mouth and lips and commence **EAR (DO NOT inhale casualty's expired air)**

1 **Determine type of poisoning:**
   - if casualty conscious, try to determine type of poison taken.

2 ☎ *Call 13 11 26 for Poisons Information Centre.*

3 **Call fire brigade if area contaminated with smoke, gases or fumes.**

4 **Monitor airway and breathing:**
   - if casualty loses consciousness, follow DRABC.

DRABC

5 ☎ *Call 000 for an ambulance.*

HEAD INJURY

1 **Monitor breathing and pulse:**
   • if casualty unconscious, follow DRABC
   • keep casualty's airway open with fingers (if face badly injured).

   DRABC

2 **Support head and neck:**
   • support casualty's head and neck during movement in case the spine is injured.

3 **Control bleeding:**
   • place sterile pad or dressing over wound
   • apply direct pressure to wound **unless** you suspect a skull fracture
   • if blood or fluid comes from ear, secure a sterile dressing lightly in place and allow to drain.

4 **Lie casualty down:**
   • place casualty in comfortable position with head and shoulders slightly raised
   • be prepared to turn casualty onto side if they vomit
   • clear the airway quickly after vomiting.

5 ☎ *Call 000 for an ambulance.*

Spinal Injury

1 **Swift immobilisation is highest priority:**
- do not move casualty unless in danger.

2 **Check breathing and pulse:**
- if casualty unconscious, follow DRABC.

3 **Support casualty's head and neck at all times:**
- place hands on side of head until other support arranged

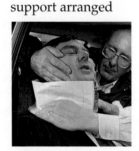

- apply a cervical or improvised collar to minimise neck movement.

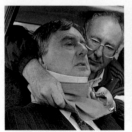 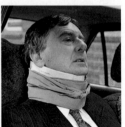

4 **Give reassurance:**
- calm casualty.

5 ☎ *Call 000 for an ambulance.*

EYE INJURY

1 **Support casualty's head:**
- support casualty's head to keep it as still as possible
- ask casualty to try not to move eyes.

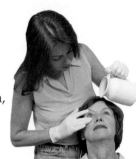

2 **Flush eye with cool, flowing water:**
- if chemical or heat burn, or smoke in eyes, flush with water.

3 **Place dressing over eye:**
- place a sterile pad or dressing over injured eye
- ask casualty to hold this in place
- bandage dressing in place, covering injured eye
- if embedded object in eye, lie casualty on back, place pad around object and bandage in place.

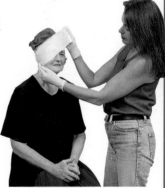

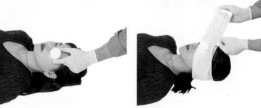

4 ☎ *Call 000 for an ambulance.*

FRACTURES, DISLOCATIONS, SPRAINS AND STRAINS

Fracture and dislocation

- pain at or near the site of the injury

- difficult or impossible normal movement

- loss of power

- deformity or abnormal mobility

- tenderness

- swelling

- discolouration and bruising

FRACTURES AND DISLOCATIONS

1 Follow DRABC.

2 Control any bleeding and cover any wounds.

3 Check for fractures:
- open, closed or complicated.

4 Ask casualty not to move injured part.

5 Immobilise fracture:
- use broad bandages (where possible) to prevent movement at joints above and below the fracture
- support the limb, carefully passing bandages under the natural hollows of the body
- place a padded splint along the injured limb (under leg for fractured kneecap)

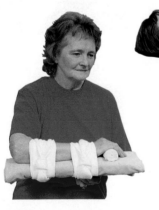

- place padding between the splint and the natural contours of the body and secure tightly
- check that bandages not too tight (or too loose) every 15 minutes.

NOTE

If collarbone fractured, support arm on injured side in a St John sling.

If dislocation of a joint is suspected, rest, elevate and apply ice to joint.

It can be difficult for a first aider to tell whether the injury is a fracture, dislocation, sprain or strain. If in doubt, always treat as a fracture.

6 **For leg fracture, immobilise foot and ankle:**
• use figure of eight bandage.

7 **Watch for signs of loss of circulation to foot or hand.**

8 ☎ *Call 000 for an ambulance.*

SPRAINS AND STRAINS

1 **Follow DRABC.**

2 **Follow RICE management plan:**
R—rest
I—ice
C—compression
E—elevation.

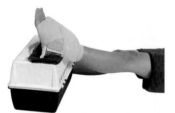 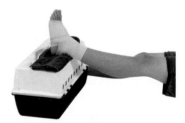

3 Seek medical aid.

HEAT-INDUCED CONDITIONS

- feeling hot, exhausted and weak

- persistent headache

- thirst and nausea

- giddiness and faintness

- fatigue

- rapid breathing and shortness of breath

- pale, cool, clammy skin

- rapid, weak pulse

Additional symptoms

- high body temperature

- flushed skin

- irritability and mental confusion may progress to seizure and unconsciousness

WARNING

Heatstroke may develop.

HEAT EXHAUSTION

1 **Lie casualty down:**
- move casualty to lie down in a cool place with circulating air.

2 **Loosen tight clothing:**
- remove unnecessary garments.

3 **Sponge with cold water.**

4 **Give fluids to drink.**

5 **Seek medical aid:**
- if casualty vomits
- if casualty does not recover promptly.

HEATSTROKE

1 **Follow DRABC.**

DRABC

2 **Apply cold packs or ice:**
- apply to neck, groin and armpits.

3 **Cover with wet sheet.**

4 **If conscious, give fluids.**

HYPOTHERMIA

SIGNS & SYMPTOMS

When body temperature falls, early warning signs may include:

- feeling cold

- shivering

- clumsiness and slurred speech

- apathy and irrational behaviour

- heart rate may slow

WARNING

☎ *Call 000 for an ambulance* if level of consciousness declines, shivering stops, pulse is difficult to find. Use any other available forms of warming except direct radiant heat.

1 Follow DRABC.

2 Remove casualty to a warm, dry place.

3 Protect casualty:
- protect casualty and yourself from wind, rain, sleet, cold, and wet ground.

4 Avoid excess activity or movement.

5 Maintain casualty in horizontal position.

6 Remove wet clothing.

7 Warm casualty:
- place between blankets or in sleeping bag, and wrap in space blanket or similar.

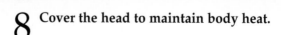

8 Cover the head to maintain body heat.

9 Give warm drinks if conscious:
- do not give alcohol.

E 31

INFANTILE CONVULSIONS

1 **During convulsions:**
  • place child on floor for safety
  • do not restrain child.

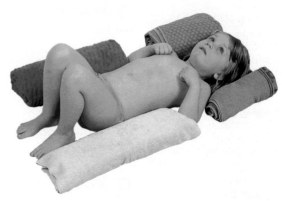

2 **After convulsions:**
  • follow DRABC
  •   turn child on side
  • remove excessive clothing or wrapping
  • seek medical aid.

DRABC

DIABETIC EMERGENCY

**Signs—
low blood sugar**

• pale

• hungry

• sweating

• weak

• confused

• aggressive

**Signs—
high blood sugar**

• thirsty

• needs to urinate

• hot dry skin

• smell of acetone
on breath

If casualty unconscious:
• follow DRABC
• ☎ *call 000 for an ambulance.*

*If casualty conscious, and signs suggest
low blood sugar:*
• give sweet food or drink (not diet, diabetic or
sugar-free drinks) every 15 minutes until casualty
recovers or medical aid arrives
• ☎ *call 000 for an ambulance.*

*If casualty conscious, and signs suggest high
blood sugar:*
• allow casualty to self-administer insulin—do
not administer it for them but assist if required
• ☎ *call 000 for an ambulance*
• give casualty sugar-free fluids to drink, if
help delayed.

NOTE: *If you are not sure which form of diabetic
emergency the casualty has, give a sweet drink. If
casualty has a high blood sugar emergency, then
giving a sweet drink will not do undue harm.*

EPILEPTIC SEIZURE

SIGNS& SYMPTOMS

Casualty may:

- suddenly cry out

- fall to ground

- have a congested and blue face and neck

- have jerky, spasmodic muscular movements

- froth at the mouth

- bite the tongue

- lose control of bladder and bowel

1 **Check breathing and pulse:**
- follow DRABC.

DRABC

2 **Protect casualty:**
- protect from injury
- do not restrict movement
- do not place anything in mouth.

3 **Manage injuries:**
- place on side as soon as possible
- manage injuries resulting from seizure
- do not disturb if casualty falls asleep
- continue to check airway, breathing and pulse.

4 **Seek medical aid if:**
- the seizure continues for more than 5 minutes
- another seizure quickly follows
- the person has been injured.

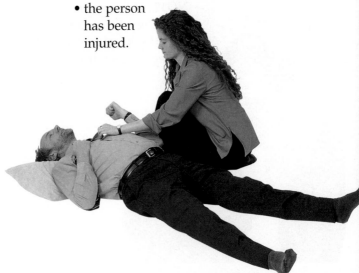

ABOUT THIS BOOK

This is the St John Ambulance Australia authorised manual for its first aid certificate courses. It may also be read as a comprehensive guide on the normal range of first aid procedures, or used as a reference as occasion may demand. **However, it must be stressed that reading this book, without attending a St John course with its practical components, does not constitute a complete first aid education.**

The initial section, Emergency First Aid—A Quick Guide, provides the essentials of first aid for the major emergencies the first aider may need to deal with. This is a ready-reference summary, not a substitute for the full coverage given in the main body of the book.

Throughout the book:

> BOXES SHADED IN BEIGE CONTAIN
> BACKGROUND INFORMATION.

> BOXES SHADED IN GREEN CONTAIN FIRST AID
> MANAGEMENT INFORMATION.

> BOXES OUTLINED IN RED CONTAIN
> SAFETY INFORMATION.

An index and a glossary are included to help the reader.

Chapter

1

The emergency situation

CONTENTS

First aid skills are based on knowledge, training and experience. First aid is help given by someone on the spot to a person who is injured or has become ill. The skills of first aid are for all.

You will acquire these skills through the information in this book and through completing a course with St John Ambulance. These skills will give you the confidence to deal with emergency situations.

In this chapter we introduce some key elements of first aid, including the St John DRABC Action Plan, and general principles for dealing with emergency situations and managing casualties. The detailed procedures for DRABC and for managing specific injuries and illnesses are given in subsequent chapters.

WHAT IS FIRST AID?

First aid is the initial care of the ill or injured. At any time, you may find yourself in a situation where someone has had an accident or is suffering from a sudden illness and needs help until a qualified health care professional, such as a doctor, registered nurse or ambulance officer, arrives.

The aims of first aid

▶ promote a safe environment
▶ preserve life
▶ prevent injury or illness from becoming worse
▶ help promote recovery
▶ provide comfort to the ill or injured

WHAT A FIRST AIDER SHOULD DO

▶ Assess the situation quickly.

▶ Identify the nature of the injury or illness as far as possible.

▶ Manage the casualty promptly and appropriately.

▶ Arrange for emergency services to attend.

▶ Stay with the casualty until able to hand over to a health care professional.

▶ Give further help if necessary.

OTHER FIRST AIDERS

The first aider who arrives first at the scene of an incident takes charge and stays in charge until handing over control. Any other first aider who arrives should offer to help the original first aider, without trying to take over control.

If you feel another first aider at the scene is more qualified to handle the situation, ask that person

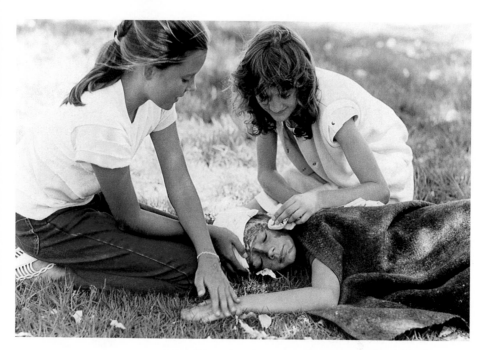

to take control. However, the most qualified person does not need to be in control, especially if another first aider already has matters well in hand.

MEDICAL AID

Medical aid is treatment by a health care professional—doctor, registered nurse or ambulance officer. Medical aid takes over from first aid when the health professional arrives at the scene of an incident. The first aider may be required to remain and assist if requested by the health care professional.

SMOKING IN RELATION TO FIRST AID

At a first aid scene, St John Ambulance Australia discourages smoking by first aiders, casualties and bystanders because of the possible presence of flammable fuel and the use of medical gases.

GETTING MEDICAL HELP FOR AN UNCONSCIOUS CASUALTY

ONE FIRST AIDER

It is vital to get help as quickly as possible. If you are the only first aider, you have to decide whether to start resuscitation or go for help first. To do this:

ASSESS THE CASUALTY

Unconscious and breathing

1 Place in recovery position *(see p. 31).*

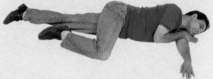

2 ☎ *Call 000 for an ambulance.*

Unconscious and not breathing (see note)

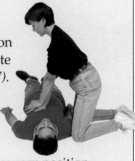

1 Give resuscitation for 1 minute *(see p. 36–7).*

2 Place in recovery position *(see p. 31).*

3 ☎ *Call 000 for an ambulance.*

Note:
- *if a non-breathing casualty is an adult, go for help immediately unless casualty is obviously injured, or it is a drowning incident*
- *if the casualty is an infant or child, give one minute of resuscitation and take them with you when you go for help; continue resuscitation on the way*

MORE THAN ONE FIRST AIDER

ASSESS THE CASUALTY

1 Start resuscitation if required.

2 Second first aider ☎ *Call 000 for an ambulance.*

THE EMERGENCY SITUATION

In an emergency, your involvement as a trained first aider may be crucial. Sometimes, bystanders are reluctant to act at an emergency because they may be unsure of what to do. Therefore, the attitude of the first aider is very important in ensuring that time is not lost in getting emergency care to the casualty and in administering the necessary first aid.

The calm, controlled manner of a confident first aider may be all it takes to give confidence to others to ensure that the emergency is handled effectively, efficiently and speedily.

YOU CAN ALWAYS DO SOMETHING TO HELP

- **Ensure safety** of yourself, bystanders and the casualty
- **Be alert** to possible dangers
- ☎ *Call 000 for an ambulance.*
- **Communicate** effectively to calm and reassure the casualty
- **Gather information** from the casualty, bystanders and anyone else who can help
- **Provide necessary** information to emergency personnel

- **Organise bystanders to**
  - ☎ *call 000 for an ambulance.*
  - ensure the safety of the accident scene
  - redirect traffic or warn oncoming traffic if a road accident has occurred
  - comfort the casualty
  - help obtain necessary supplies

Note: If using a mobile phone, use the number 000 to call for help–if this does not work try 112.

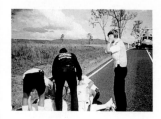

Having an emergency action plan will mean that any initial confusion you may feel can be overcome. It will help ensure that you:
- remain calm and don't panic;
- are aware of and can respond to the safety needs of the emergency scene;

▶ are able to assess which casualty's needs take first aid priority;
▶ deal with any injuries in order of severity and how life-threatening they are
▶ know when and how to move a casualty
▶ gather the information which will be needed by emergency services

SAFETY AT THE SCENE

The emergency scene must be made safe for everyone—yourself, bystanders and the casualty. You will need to determine if:
▶ there is any continuing danger (e.g. a fallen powerline)
▶ anyone's life is in immediate danger (e.g. from a fire or flammable materials)

Leave dangerous situations for emergency personnel to deal with as they have the training and equipment to do so.

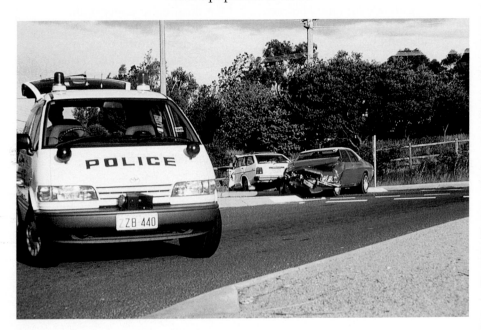

However, after assessing the situation, remove the danger or prevent new dangers whenever possible. For example, if a child has received an electric shock at home, it should be possible to turn off the electricity immediately at the power point or at the main switchboard.

At the scene of a car accident, you can position other cars with their hazard lights flashing to warn oncoming traffic of the danger. At night it is also recommended that headlights are switched on to illuminate the scene.

If at any time you suspect the scene is unsafe, it is better to wait and watch until emergency personnel arrive than to place yourself and others in danger.

THE CASUALTY

You may feel uncertain about touching someone who is a stranger, who is of a different age group, race, or sex, or is from your workplace.

Your ability to deal with the emergency and perhaps save the person's life will depend on your ability to put aside these concerns and deal with the emergency in the best way you can.

Casualty behaviour

A casualty's behaviour may also cause you to be hesitant about giving first aid. The casualty may be acting strangely or be uncooperative. Sometimes a casualty may act in an offensive manner as a result of the injury or illness, or because of stress or the influence of alcohol or other drugs. Attempt to establish a rapport with the casualty by introducing yourself and asking the casualty's name.

If the casualty's behaviour prevents you from giving help, there are still things you can do:

▶ make sure someone has called the appropriate emergency services

▶ manage bystanders

▶ try to reassure and calm the casualty

If at any time the casualty's behaviour poses a threat to you, withdraw from the scene. If necessary, monitor from a safe distance and make sure other bystanders are safe.

Disease transmission

An awareness of disease transmission is extremely important, especially in relation to hepatitis and HIV/AIDS. The actual risk of transmission in first aid is extremely low. Nevertheless, the safety procedures in any emergency situation involve taking general steps to protect against infection and reduce the risk.

By taking precautions—such as wearing disposable gloves—to prevent direct contact with bodily fluids while giving first aid, and by washing thoroughly straight after giving first aid, you are observing 'best practice' health care. If you do come into contact with a casualty's bodily fluids, seek medical advice as soon as possible.

Nature of the injury or illness

Sometimes the nature of the injury or illness, unpleasant smells, or the sight of blood, vomit, or torn skin may be disconcerting or distressing. This is natural; even salaried ambulance officers and doctors sometimes experience these reactions. If you need to prepare yourself to act, turning away and taking a few deep breaths while telling yourself of the importance of your first aid skills will help to put you in the necessary frame of mind.

USE OF BYSTANDERS

Emergencies attract a lot of attention so there may be many people standing around watching. To give the casualty the safest care possible, only those people really needed should be at the scene. These include:

▶ any witnesses to the incident
▶ relatives and close friends of the casualty
▶ any bystanders you ask to stay to help

Everyone else should be asked to move well away. If necessary, a bystander could control the crowd.

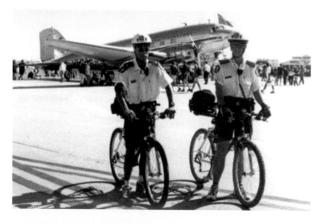

Always look for bystanders who can help in some way or who may be able to tell you what happened. A bystander may be able to:

▶ tell you exactly how an accident happened
▶ give you information on relevant medical problems or allergies
▶ help make the scene safe
▶ keep the area free of unnecessary traffic
▶ call paramedics, medical officers or local authorities (e.g. to have power turned off)
▶ help provide care
▶ gather and protect the casualty's belongings

▶ find a first aid kit or alternative materials
▶ take notes
▶ ease concerns of the casualty's relatives and friends
▶ help protect the privacy of the casualty

INFORMATION REQUIRED BY EMERGENCY SERVICES

When ringing emergency services:
▶ make sure you have all the necessary information before speaking to the operator
▶ keep messages brief and accurate
▶ ensure messages are not given too quickly, are clear and can be easily understood

PRIORITIES OF MANAGEMENT

In dealing with an accident, illness or any other situation that requires the help of a first aider, it is important to determine which injuries or conditions are most in need of your attention. In the primary assessment, determine whether:
▶ casualty is conscious
▶ airway is clear and open
▶ casualty is breathing
▶ casualty has a pulse
▶ there is any bleeding

Unconsciousness is a life-threatening condition

If casualty is unconscious:
▶ the airway may be blocked if tongue has relaxed and fallen to back of throat (causing breathing to stop and, soon after, the heart to stop beating)
▶ there is risk of choking as casualty has no ability to swallow, or to cough out any object
▶ the capacity for self-protection from potential dangers (e.g. traffic, fire, a collapsing building, drowning) may be lost

CALLING EMERGENCY SERVICES

1 ☎ *Call 000 for an ambulance.*

2 Ask for the ambulance service (ambulance will call other services if required).

3 Give the exact place of the accident with directions.

4 Give the number of casualties.

5 Give an indication of the type and extent of injuries.

6 State if any other emergency services are required.

7 Give the telephone number of the phone you are using.

8 Ask the likely time of arrival of the ambulance service.

In a city or town, give:	In a rural area, give:	If a road accident, give:
• street number • street • landmarks (e.g. cross street) • suburb • city/town	• distance from intersection/landmark/roadside number • road • area • nearest city/town • landmark	• number of people involved • is anybody trapped? • are powerlines involved? • other hazards

Describe location

Name of district, suburb, etc: *NUNAWADING*

Name of street, road, highway, etc: *Maroondah Hwy*

Nearest cross street (suburban): *Springvale Road*

Distance from town or major landmark (country) .... kms

North ☐   South ☐   East ☐   West ☐

of ....(describe town or landmark)

Give accident details

Number of people hurt *3 (2 adults, 1 infant)*

Time of accident (if known) *3.15 am approx*

Time this message written *3.21 am*

Notes *Truck and family sedan have collided on corner — Big petrol spill. Infant critical. Melway 48 F9*

11

When there is more than one casualty, you will have to assess quickly which casualty takes priority. This will mean assessing which injuries are the most serious and which of these need the most immediate attention. A noisy, demanding casualty may be a lower priority than the silent casualty who may have a blocked airway.

The decisions you make about which casualty most urgently needs help may be influenced by factors not related to their injuries. If one of the seriously injured casualties is trapped in a car, it may be difficult for you to give other than minimal first aid. In such a situation, you may have to decide that someone else who is not as seriously injured has priority.

MOVEMENT OF A CASUALTY

Unless absolutely necessary do not move a casualty until medical aid arrives. Moving a casualty unnecessarily may lead to further injury.

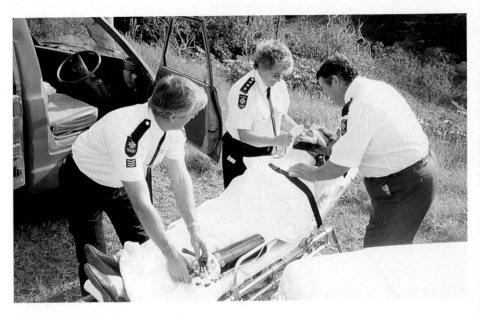

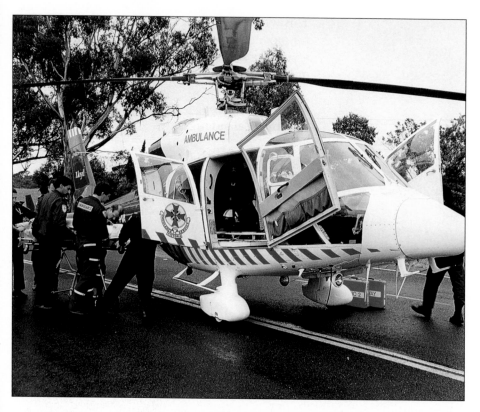

If the casualty's life is endangered (e.g. by the risk of an explosion, drowning, or collapse of a burning building), remove the casualty from the scene by the quickest and safest means available, regardless of injuries or the manner in which removal must be made. **If a neck or spinal injury is suspected, support for the neck must be provided before moving** *(see p. 162).*

Before you act, consider:
- the dangerous conditions at the scene
- the casualty's size
- your own health and physical ability
- if there are others who can help
- the casualty's condition

This will help you decide the best method to use for moving the casualty, whether you need assistance and whether other aids such as a chair or blanket are needed.

When injuries appear to be serious or extensive, seek medical aid urgently.

Road or air ambulance is the preferred method of transporting the seriously injured casualty. Improvised transport may endanger the casualty's chance of survival and should only be used if no ambulance is available.

After the Emergency

In first aid we prepare ourselves for all types of emergency situations, but we don't always think about what happens after the casualty has left our care.

Once you have handed the casualty over to the ambulance or a doctor, there may be a number of practical things that need attention. These may include cleaning up the accident scene, correcting any unsafe conditions that caused the accident, or making a report (e.g. in a workplace).

POST-TRAUMATIC STRESS

Although life seems to go back to normal, many people think back over a stressful event and try to evaluate what more they could have done. The more serious the incident, the more you are likely to think about it.

This is completely normal. But if it continues for weeks or begins to affect your day-to-day life, you may be experiencing post-traumatic stress.

Post-traumatic stress is a possible reaction to a stressful event. It needs to be dealt with, as it can affect your relationships, your concentration and your peace of mind.

Go and talk to your doctor or a counsellor. They will understand what you are going through and will be able to suggest a course of action to help you deal with the effects of post-traumatic stress.

General Principles of Casualty Management

PRIORITIES

Emergencies often result in confusion. Those nearby may not know what to do first, who should take charge or how to get help. Following a sequence of actions will help ensure safe, appropriate first aid is given.

1 **DRABC and initial assessment:**
- what dangers are present to you, bystanders and the casualty?
- how many casualties are there?
- what caused the injury?
- is the casualty conscious?
- is the airway clear and open?
- is resuscitation needed *(see ch. 2)*?

2 **Phone for medical assistance:**
- ☎ *Call 000 for an ambulance.*
  OR
- send someone to phone for an ambulance.

3 **Secondary assessment:**
- question the casualty and bystanders to find out what happened
- check vital signs (level of consciousness, breathing, pulse, skin colour and temperature) and monitor every 15 minutes
- check symptoms (e.g. pain)
- check signs of injury (e.g. deformed limbs, bleeding) or of a specific medical condition (e.g. epilepsy)
- decide which injuries or conditions need care.

4 **Ongoing casualty care:**
  ▶ monitor the casualty's condition
  ▶ record details of events/situation
  ▶ stay with the casualty until medical aid arrives
  ▶ report what first aid has been given.

DRABC

The St John DRABC Action Plan is a vital aid to the first aider in casualty management.

D	for	**Danger**
R	for	**Response**
A	for	**Airway**
B	for	**Breathing**
C	for	**Circulation**

This plan helps you find out if the casualty has any life-threatening conditions and helps you give any immediately necessary first aid. The detailed implementation of DRABC is set out in chapter two, Adult Basic Life Support.

Once you have applied the principles of DRABC, and if necessary phoned for an ambulance, proceed to:
  ▶ take a history of the casualty
  ▶ monitor vital signs
  ▶ carry out a head-to-toe examination
  ▶ give first aid for injuries and illnesses that are not life-threatening

1 **History from the casualty:**
  When you are taking a history from a casualty, the aim is to find out anything that may be important about the casualty and the situation:

▶ events leading to incident—ask how the incident happened

▶ symptoms—find out casualty's symptoms (pain, nausea etc.)

▶ allergies—ask if casualty has any allergies

▶ past medical history—check for a Medic Alert bracelet or anything that could relate to the current injury or illness

▶ medication—ask if casualty has taken any medication in the last 24 hours or is on regular medication and if they have any with them

▶ last meal—ask when casualty last had anything to eat or drink.

2 Vital signs:

These show the basic condition of the casualty. Any change in the casualty's vital signs could indicate a serious change in condition. The vital signs are:

▶ level of consciousness (conscious or unconscious)

▶ breathing

▶ pulse

▶ skin colour and temperature.

Level of consciousness Ask:

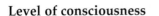

• *open your eyes*

• *what is your name?*

• *can you move your fingers?*

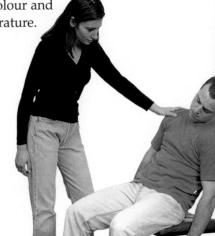

Breathing

- look for chest movements
- listen for sounds of breathing from the mouth
- feel for breath on your check

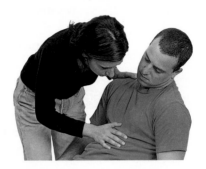

Pulse

- use index and middle fingers to find the pulse (*never use the thumb as you may feel its own pulse*)
- the radial pulse is beside the crease lines at the wrist, on the same side as thumb
- the carotid pulse is on either side of the windpipe (*only check one side at one time*)
  Note: Check brachial pulse in infants—see instructions on page 53.

Skin colour and temperature

- use the back of the hand to assess skin temperature
- is the skin pale? bluish? clammy? wet?

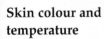

19

3 Head-to-toe examination:
Note: In carrying out a head-to-toe examination, be especially sensitive to the age, sex and race of the person you are examining.

1 Examine head
- check for bruising, blood and swelling

2 Check face
- check eyes (compare size of pupils, look for bruising, cuts and swelling)
- compare one side of face to the other

3 Check neck
- check for injuries (bruising, cuts, etc.)
- check collarbones (breakages, bruising, etc.)

4 Check shoulders, arms and hands
- check shoulder joint and shoulderblade
- check full length of each arm
- check hand and each finger for bruising, swelling, cuts, breaks and feeling

5 Check chest
- does it expand easily and evenly?
- does breathing cause pain?
- check for injuries (bruising, cuts, etc.)

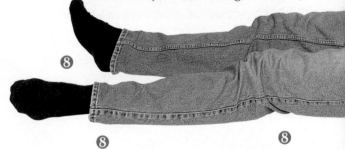

⑧

⑧   ⑧

6 Check abdomen
- is it tender—does a gentle press on the abdomen cause pain?
- check for injuries (bruising, cuts, etc.)

7 Check pelvis and buttocks
- push tops of hips towards each other—does this cause pain?
- check for injuries (bruising, cuts, etc.)
- check for evidence of wet pants or blood from genital area

8 Check legs, ankles and feet
- check right along each leg for bruising, swelling, cuts, breaks, and abnormal alignment
- check foot and each toe for bruising, swelling, cuts, breaks and feeling

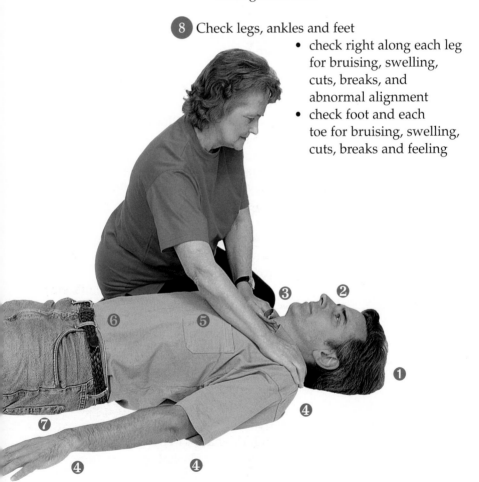

THE UNCONSCIOUS OR PARTIALLY CONSCIOUS CASUALTY

In any emergency there is the possibility that a casualty will be unconscious or partially conscious (the latter is often referred to as an 'altered conscious state').

If a person is unconscious or partially conscious, it indicates that something serious and possibly life-threatening is wrong. The brain is the controlling organ of the body and regulates all body functions. Any injury serious enough to alter the consciousness of the casualty may have caused damage to the brain.

Unconsciousness or an altered conscious state can be caused by:

▶ direct injury to or illness affecting the brain as a result of
  • head injury
  • a stroke
  • fits/seizures
  • meningitis

▶ lack of oxygen to the brain as a result of
  • cardiac arrest
  • irregular heartbeat
  • shock
  • severe respiratory problems including asthma
  • a blocked airway
  • smoke inhalation

▶ poisons and toxic products in the blood as a result of
  • diabetes
  • kidney and/or liver failure
  • overdose of alcohol or other drug

Usually the loss or partial loss of consciousness is temporary. However, a casualty may be left permanently brain damaged by any of these conditions.

Good assessment and management of an unconscious or semi-conscious casualty can not only save life but can make all the difference to the future quality of life in survivors.

The level of consciousness may indicate the amount of damage to the brain. Until medical aid arrives, the level of consciousness must be assessed regularly, every 15 minutes, and preferably recorded.

Management

The general management of an unconscious person is the same, whatever the cause of unconsciousness. The casualty needs:
- protection from danger (e.g. oncoming traffic)
- to be in recovery position
- a clear airway
- treatment of other injuries (e.g. fractures splinted, wounds covered)
- ☎ *call 000 for an ambulance.*

EXAMINATION OF AN UNCONSCIOUS CASUALTY
CHECKLIST

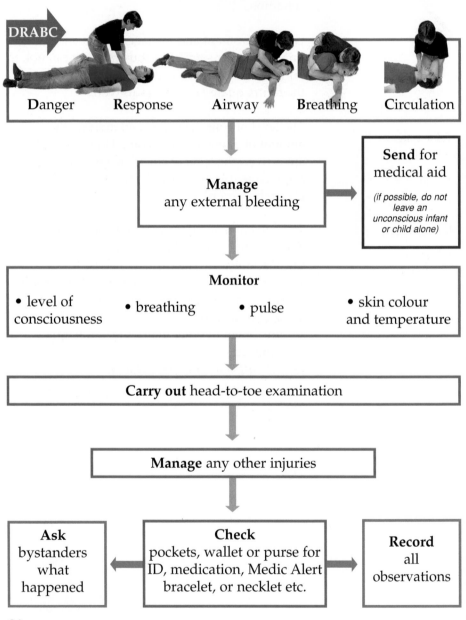

DRABC

Danger   **Response**   **Airway**   **Breathing**   **Circulation**

Manage
any external bleeding

Send for medical aid

(if possible, do not leave an unconscious infant or child alone)

Monitor

• level of consciousness   • breathing   • pulse   • skin colour and temperature

Carry out head-to-toe examination

Manage any other injuries

Ask bystanders what happened

Check pockets, wallet or purse for ID, medication, Medic Alert bracelet, or necklet etc.

Record all observations

Adult basic
life support

If you are faced with an emergency in which there is a life-threatening situation, what you do in the first few minutes is critical. Not only can it mean the difference between life and death, but it could also influence the casualty's full recovery.

This chapter will explain how, if breathing has stopped, you can supply oxygen to the casualty's lungs until breathing starts again; how, if the heart has stopped beating, you can provide the necessary life support to pump oxygenated blood around the body to preserve brain function.

This chapter also discusses how to deal with the situation if a casualty goes into shock, and how to prevent this.

ADULT BASIC LIFE SUPPORT

D Danger
R Response
A Airway
B Breathing
C Circulation

Basic life support is essentially the ABC of emergency care. It is the action taken to maintain airway, breathing and circulation, and thereby life itself, in the hope that the natural function of the lungs and heart will be restored.

When a casualty stops breathing (respiratory arrest), the heart can continue to pump blood for several minutes only. Early intervention to restore the casualty's breathing may prevent the heart stopping (cardiac arrest). If cardiac arrest does occur, cardiopulmonary resuscitation (CPR) must be swiftly applied or the casualty is sure to die. **CPR is the combination of expired air resuscitation (EAR) and external cardiac compression (ECC).**

There are three main actions in providing basic life support.

1 **Maintaining an airway**—this may involve having to move an obstruction, such as the tongue, from the airway.

2 **Giving expired air resuscitation (EAR)**— using your breath to inflate a casualty's lungs by breathing into casualty's mouth.

3 **Giving external cardiac compression (ECC)** —external chest compressions carried out in a rhythmical fashion; always combined with expired air resuscitation.

These simple techniques will either restart normal heart action or maintain circulation sufficient to preserve brain function until specialised assessment and treatment are available.

CHAIN OF SURVIVAL

Measures to maximise a casualty's chances of
survival, particularly when the heart stops, have
to be taken immediately. This 'chain of survival'
is the key to improving the survival rate from
cardiac and respiratory arrest in our community.
Time is of the essence!

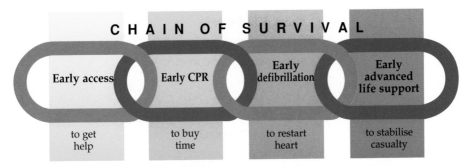

CHAIN OF SURVIVAL

Early access	Early CPR	Early defibrillation	Early advanced life support
to get help	to buy time	to restart heart	to stabilise casualty

WHAT IS THE CHAIN OF SURVIVAL?

Early access

The ambulance must be called immediately to
ensure that early defibrillation and advanced life
support can commence without delay.

Early CPR

If CPR is begun within 4 minutes of the heart
stopping, oxygenation of the vital organs (such as
the brain) is maintained.

Early defibrillation

If CPR is given within 4 minutes and defibrillation
within 8–12 minutes, there is a significantly
improved chance of survival.

**Early advanced
cardiac life support**

Definitive treatment by the ambulance service,
such as giving medication and stabilising the
airway, may increase chances of survival even
further.

27

THE DRABC ACTION PLAN

D check for **DANGER**
- to you
- to others
- to casualty

R check **RESPONSE**
- is casualty conscious?
- is casualty unconscious?

A check **AIRWAY**
- is airway clear of objects?
- is airway open?

B check for **BREATHING**
- is chest rising and falling?
- can you hear breathing?
- can you feel breath on your cheek?

C check **CIRCULATION**
- can you feel a pulse?
- can you see any obvious signs of life?

D DANGER

In every emergency situation, it is important to see if there are any conditions that may be an immediate threat to life. It is most important to make sure the area is safe for both the casualty and yourself. You are no help to the casualty if you become a casualty yourself. Once you have made sure the area is safe, you can go ahead with assessing the casualty.

R RESPONSE
(CONSCIOUSNESS)

The next step is to determine if the casualty is conscious:

▶ ask casualty's name
▶ gently shake casualty's shoulder
OR

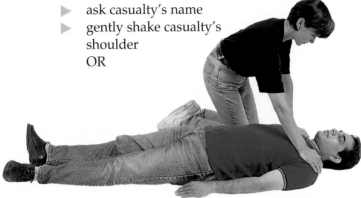

▶ ask casualty to squeeze your hands (both sides should be tried if a stroke is suspected)

A response indicates that the casualty is conscious and can be left in the position in which you found them (provided there is no further danger). Then follow the steps below.

1 Manage any life-threatening injuries that need immediate attention.

2 Manage other injuries (if left unattended, these may become life-threatening).

3 Get help if injuries require it.

4 Calm the casualty.

No response indicates that the casualty is unconscious and it is important to get help as quickly as possible as unconsciousness is a life-threatening condition *(see p. 4)*.

1 Shout for help or send someone for help.

2 Consider going to get help yourself if you are alone, but only if the casualty is in the recovery position, and the airway is clear.

A AIRWAY

It is essential to the casualty's chance of survival to ensure that the airway is clear so that breathing is possible. Turn the casualty onto side, into the recovery position. Ensure neck is well supported if a neck or spine injury is suspected *(see p. 162)*.

Clear airway

1 Open the mouth and clear any foreign objects with your fingers. Only remove dentures if they are loose or broken.

2 Tilt the head back gently and slightly down.

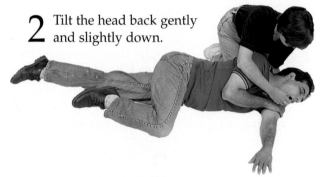

Obstruction of the airway may be caused by:
▶ the tongue
▶ solid or semi-solid material such as food, vomit, blood or a foreign body
▶ laryngeal spasm
▶ swelling or injury of the airway

Open airway

1 Place your hand high on the casualty's forehead.

2 Support the chin with your other hand.

(continued p. 32)

THE RECOVERY POSITION

1 Kneel beside casualty.

2 Lift nearer leg at knee so it is fully bent upwards.

3 Place nearer arm across chest.

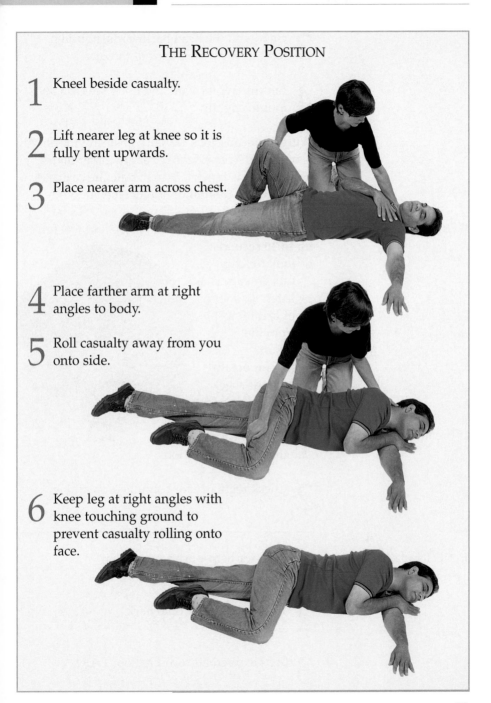

4 Place farther arm at right angles to body.

5 Roll casualty away from you onto side.

6 Keep leg at right angles with knee touching ground to prevent casualty rolling onto face.

3 Gently tilt the head backwards, to bring tongue away from back of throat.

4 Lift the jaw forward and open the casualty's mouth slightly.

With an unconscious casualty, ensuring the airway is open takes precedence over any other injury. However, it is important to handle the casualty gently with a minimum of movement.

B BREATHING

To check for breathing, look, listen and feel for **up to 10 seconds:**

> look for chest movements
> listen for sounds of breathing from the mouth
> feel for breath on your cheek

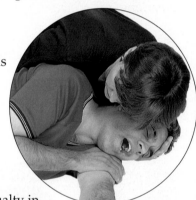

If breathing

1 Leave the casualty in the recovery position.

2 Check regularly for continued breathing.

If NOT breathing

1 Send for help—use a bystander.

2 Turn the casualty onto back.

3 Start expired air resuscitation (EAR).

EXPIRED AIR RESUSCITATION (EAR) (MOUTH-TO-MOUTH RESUSCITATION)

Expired air resuscitation (EAR) is used to breathe air into the casualty to provide the oxygen needed for survival. The air you breathe out of your lungs contains about 16% oxygen. This is more than enough to keep someone alive. *EAR alone is given to those who are not breathing but still have a pulse.*

1 Turn the casualty onto back.

2 Ensure head tilt and chin lift.

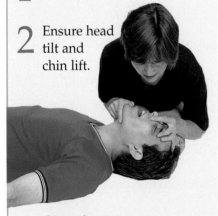

3 Open the airway:
 • place your hand on the casualty's forehead and pinch soft part of the nose closed with the index finger and thumb, or seal nose with your cheek
 • open the casualty's mouth and maintain chin lift.

4 Take a breath and place your lips on the casualty's mouth, ensuring a good seal.

5 Blow steadily into the casualty's mouth for about 1.5–2 seconds:
 • watch for chest to rise.

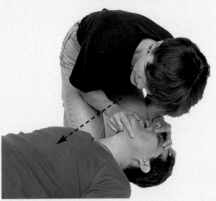

6 Maintain head tilt and chin lift.

7 Turn your mouth away from the casualty, watch for chest to fall, and listen and feel for signs of air being expelled.

8 Take another breath and repeat the sequence to give at least 2 effective breaths (i.e. 2 breaths in which the casualty's chest both rises and falls).

EXPIRED AIR RESUSCITATION *CONT.*

9   Check pulse (circulation).

If pulse present:

10 Continue EAR at 1 breath every 4 seconds (15 breaths per minute).

11 Check pulse about every minute.

If you have trouble achieving an effective breath (i.e. casualty's chest fails to rise and fall), recheck:
▶ mouth—remove any obstruction
▶ adequate head tilt and chin lift

Give up to 5 breaths to achieve at least 2 effective breaths. Even if unsuccessful, move on to assessment for circulation (pulse).

C   CIRCULATION

To assess for signs of circulation:

1 Check if carotid (neck) pulse present.

2 Look for any movement, including swallowing or breathing.

3 Observe colour of skin on face.

Take no more than 10 seconds to do this.

How to Check Pulse

To feel for pulse:

- use the pads of your fingers (NOT the thumb or fingertips)
- to find carotid pulse place your fingers in the groove on either side of the windpipe (neck), but not on both sides at the same time

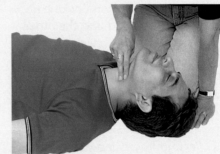

OR

- the radial pulse can be felt at the wrist

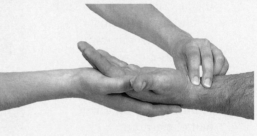

If there are signs of circulation

1   Continue EAR at 1 breath every 4 seconds (15 breaths per minute).

2   Recheck for signs of circulation about every minute.

3   If casualty starts to breathe sufficiently on own, turn onto side into the recovery position.

4   Check the casualty's condition and be ready to turn onto back and restart EAR if breathing stops.

No signs of circulation (or you are unsure)

Start cardiopulmonary resuscitation (CPR).

CARDIOPULMONARY RESUSCITATION (CPR)

1 Kneel beside casualty, one knee level with head and the other with casualty's chest.

2 Locate lower half of breastbone (sternum):
- find groove at the neck between collarbones
- find lower end of sternum by running a finger along the last rib to centre of body
- extend thumbs equal distances to meet in middle of sternum
- keep thumb of one hand in position and place heel of other hand on lower half of sternum.

3 Place heel of other hand on top of first.

4 Interlock fingers of both hands and raise fingers to ensure that pressure is not applied over casualty's ribs, upper abdomen or bottom part of sternum.

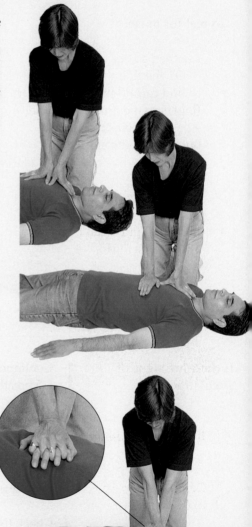

5 Position yourself vertically above casualty's chest.

6 With your arms straight, press down on the sternum to depress it about 5 cms.

9 After 15 chest compressions, tilt head and lift chin.

10 Give 2 effective breaths.

11 Return your hands immediately to correct position on sternum.

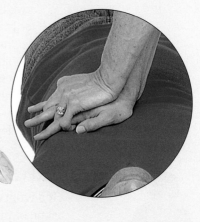

7 Release the pressure.

8 Repeat compressions at a rate of 80–100 times a minute.

Note: Compression and release should take equal amounts of time.

12 Give 15 further compressions.

13 Continue compressions and breaths in a ratio of 15:2 at a rate of 4 cycles per minute.

14 Check pulse about every minute.

When to stop CPR

You can stop giving CPR when:
- the casualty shows signs of life
- qualified help arrives
- you are physically unable to continue

After breathing and circulation have been restored

1 Turn the casualty to the recovery position.

2 Call medical aid as soon as possible (if not done already).

3 Complete an orderly casualty assessment for bleeding and other injuries noting tenderness, swelling, wounds or deformity in the following order:
- head, face and neck
- shoulders, arms and hands
- chest
- abdomen
- pelvis and buttocks
- legs, ankles and feet

PREGNANT CASUALTY

If a woman requiring CPR is in an advanced state of pregnancy:

1 Position her on back with shoulders flat.

2 Place padding under her right buttock to tilt pelvis to the left.

3 If there is not enough padding available to achieve a definite tilt, a second person should hold the casualty's abdomen to the left side while CPR is performed.

OTHER RESUSCITATION TECHNIQUES

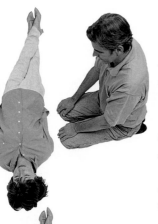

ALTERNATIVE RECOVERY POSITION

1 Kneel beside casualty.

2 Place casualty's nearer arm, palm up, under the buttocks.

3 Cross farther leg over nearer leg.

4 Place farther arm across the chest.

5 Support casualty's head and neck with one hand.

6 Grasp the casualty's farther hip with your other hand.

7 Roll casualty towards you until resting against your knees and with head resting on the ground.

8 Support casualty in this position until airway and breathing have been checked.

9 Place casualty's hand under cheek.

10 Bend upper leg at a right angle to the body.

11 Remove farther arm from under the body to ensure a stable position.

EXPIRED AIR RESUSCITATION (EAR) ALTERNATIVE METHODS

Mouth-to-nose method

The mouth-to-nose method is used when:
▶ the jaw and/or teeth are broken
▶ the jaws are tightly clenched
▶ resuscitating in deep water
▶ resuscitating an infant or small child when your mouth can cover the casualty's nose and mouth together

In order to carry out EAR using this method:

1 Kneel beside the casualty.

2 Keep the casualty's head tilted back.

3 Close the casualty's mouth.

4 Place your thumb on the lower lip to keep the casualty's mouth closed.

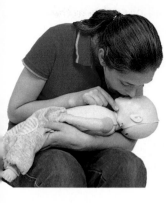

5 Support the jaw.

6 Take a deep breath and open your mouth wide.

7 Seal your mouth around the casualty's nose (infant—mouth and nose) without compressing the soft part.

8 Blow into the casualty's nose (infant—mouth and nose).

9 Remove your mouth after blowing in and allow the casualty's mouth to open by removing your thumb to allow exhalation.

Mouth-to-mask method

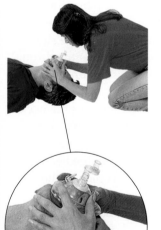

The mouth-to-mask method, using a resuscitation mask, avoids mouth-to-mouth contact between the first aider and the casualty. This is especially appropriate if the casualty has vomited, if blood is present or if the casualty is inebriated. However, resuscitation should not be delayed by attempts to obtain a mask. (An appropriate face mask is provided in the St John Ambulance Australia Communicable Diseases Protection Pack.)

In order to carry out EAR using this method:

1 Kneel—*either* beside the casualty's head *or* at the casualty's head, facing the feet.

2 Tilt the jaw slightly upwards using both hands, to maintain an open airway and to hold the mask in place.

3 Place narrow end of mask on bridge of nose (apply mask firmly to achieve an effective seal).

41

4 Take a deep breath and blow through the mouthpiece of the mask.

5 Remove your mouth to allow exhalation.

6 Turn your head to listen and feel for the escape of air.

7 If the chest does not rise, recheck head tilt, jaw support and mask seal.

8 Maintain breathing cycle.

Mouth-to-stoma method

A laryngectomee is a person who has had the larynx (voice box) removed. This is usually done as part of the treatment for cancer, but sometimes after burns, injury or infection. Removal of the larynx, total or partial, results in the person breathing through a hole (stoma) in the windpipe in the front of the neck. Some breathe only through the stoma (total neck breathers) while others breathe through stoma, mouth and nose (partial neck breathers).

A cravat, scarf or other fabric filter over the neck may alert the rescuer to the possible presence of a stoma. A stoma will be more obvious when the casualty is on the back for EAR and the head is put into backward tilt. If a tube is seen in the stoma, always leave it in place to keep the hole open for breathing and resuscitation.

In order to carry out EAR using this method:

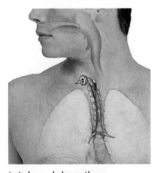

total neck breather

1 Support the jaw with the head in backward tilt to make it easier for you to seal your mouth over the stoma.

2 Take a deep breath and blow through the stoma.

3 If the chest fails to rise, this may be due to:
 ▶ a poor seal over the stoma
 ▶ the casualty being a partial neck breather, so air is escaping from mouth and nose
 ▶ a blocked stoma or tube—do not remove the blocked tube but blow harder; use lateral chest thrust *(see ch. 19)* in an attempt to dislodge the obstruction.

For a partial neck breather

1 Place one hand over the side of the casualty's face, sealing the nostrils with index and middle fingers.

2 Use the thumb to press the chin upwards and backwards, sealing the lips.

3 Take a deep breath and blow through the stoma.

4 When the chest rises, lift the fingers sealing the nose and mouth and listen for escaping air from nostrils and stoma. In a noisy environment this may be hard to hear.

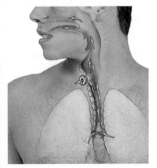

partial neck breather

SHOCK

A casualty's physical injuries may not appear to be severe but may result in life-threatening consequences associated with shock.

What is shock?

If the circulatory system fails, insufficient oxygen reaches the vital organs and the tissues of which they are composed. This triggers a series of responses that leads to the condition known as shock.

What causes shock?

If the heart fails to do its work (as in a heart attack), or the volume of blood circulating around the body is reduced (as a result of bleeding, or fluid loss from severe diarrhoea, vomiting or burns), the cells quickly become depleted of oxygen. This causes shock at the cellular level and produces the signs of shock in the whole body. This can be particularly serious in children and the elderly. A spinal cord injury can also result in shock.

Immediately after injury, there may be little evidence of shock. The signs and symptoms may develop progressively, depending on:
- the severity of the injury
- continuation of fluid loss
- effectiveness of management

INITIAL SHOCK
Signs and symptoms
- pale face, fingernails and lips
- cold, clammy skin
- faintness or dizziness
- nausea
- anxiety

SEVERE SHOCK
Signs and symptoms
- restlessness
- thirst

▶ weak, rapid pulse
▶ rapid breathing
▶ drowsiness, confusion or unconsciousness
▶ extremities become bluish in colour

MANAGEMENT OF SHOCK

1 Follow DRABC and control severe bleeding.

8 Maintain body warmth but do not heat casualty.

2 Reassure the casualty.

3 ☎ *Call 000 for an ambulance.*

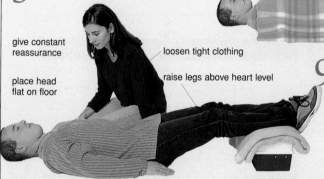

check pulse regularly

observe breathing rate and skin colour

cover with a blanket to maintain body temperature

give constant reassurance

loosen tight clothing

place head flat on floor

raise legs above heart level

9 If the casualty complains of thirst, moisten lips, but DO NOT give anything to eat or drink.

4 Raise the casualty's legs (unless fractured) above the level of the heart.

10 Monitor and record breathing and pulse at regular intervals.

5 Dress any wounds or burns.

11 Maintain a clear and open airway.

6 Immobilise any fractures.

7 Loosen any tight clothing.

12 Place casualty in recovery position if there is breathing difficulty, if vomiting is likely, or if the casualty becomes unconscious.

LIFE SUPPORT ACTION OPTIONS
(single first aider)

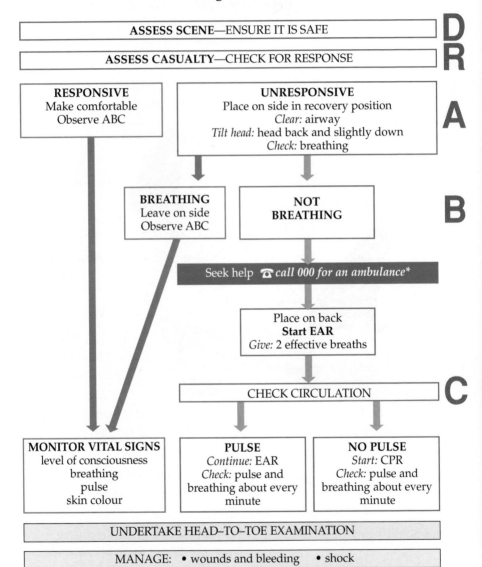

ASSESS SCENE—ENSURE IT IS SAFE	**D**
ASSESS CASUALTY—CHECK FOR RESPONSE	**R**

RESPONSIVE
Make comfortable
Observe ABC

UNRESPONSIVE
Place on side in recovery position
Clear: airway
Tilt head: head back and slightly down
Check: breathing

A

BREATHING
Leave on side
Observe ABC

NOT BREATHING

B

Seek help ☎ *call 000 for an ambulance**

Place on back
Start EAR
Give: 2 effective breaths

CHECK CIRCULATION

C

MONITOR VITAL SIGNS
level of consciousness
breathing
pulse
skin colour

PULSE
Continue: EAR
Check: pulse and
breathing about every
minute

NO PULSE
Start: CPR
Check: pulse and
breathing about every
minute

UNDERTAKE HEAD–TO–TOE EXAMINATION

MANAGE: • wounds and bleeding • shock

* Note: If the cause of collapse is near drowning, give 5 initial breaths then continue resuscitation for 1 minute before going for help. If a child or infant, take with you if possible and continue resuscitation: if an adult, place in recovery position.

Infant and child basic life support

Children can become ill quickly and are very prone to accidents. They may respond more dramatically than adults to injuries and illnesses but have great powers of potential recovery.

The process of giving expired air resuscitation (EAR) and external cardiac compression (ECC) to infants and children is much the same as for adults. However, because they have smaller bodies, the rate of breaths given for infants and young children in EAR is higher than for adults, while the pressure used to give compressions in ECC is lower.

INFANT AND CHILD BASIC LIFE SUPPORT

As with adults, an infant or child who stops breathing will become unconscious because there is no oxygen reaching the brain. Lack of oxygen will also cause the heartbeat to slow down until it stops. You need to ensure the airway is clear and get air into the lungs as quickly as possible. If the heart has stopped, you need to get blood flowing to the brain again.

In determining which resuscitation technique to use, the age of the child needs to be considered. For resuscitation purposes children are classified as follows:

Infant: newborn–1 year
Young child: 1–8 years
Older child: 9–14 years

For an older child, use the same resuscitation techniques as for adults *(see ch. 2).*

Before rushing to help a child, it is necessary first to assess the situation.

DRABC Action Plan

D   DANGER

1 **Check for danger**—particularly any continuing danger (such as fire, fumes or electricity) to yourself and the child.

2 **If possible, remove the child from the danger, or the danger from the child.**

3 **Shout for help** as someone may be within earshot.

R   RESPONSE

Check immediately to determine if the child is conscious:

▸ call child's name, if known
▸ gently shake child's shoulder
▸ squeeze tip of finger

Note: Don't shake an infant or a young child.

gently shake child's shoulder

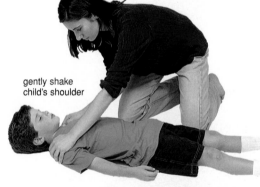

If the child is unconscious, place in the normal recovery position *(see p. 31)*. **For infants,** the most suitable recovery position is lying face down on an adult's forearm with the head supported by the hand *(see p. 50)*.

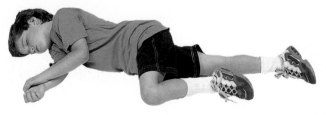

A AIRWAY

The aim is to remove any obstruction and open the airway.

Clear airway
INFANT (to 1 year)

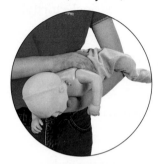

Infant recovery position

1 With infant in recovery position, clear mouth and nostrils of foreign material.

2 Place infant flat on back.

3 Tilt head back very slightly, to achieve an open airway.

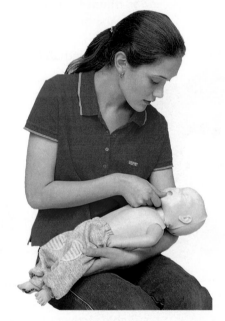

4 Lift chin to bring tongue away from back of throat.

5 Avoid pressure on soft tissue under infant's chin.

Note: Do not tilt the head if you suspect a neck injury.

Clear airway
CHILD (1–8 years)

1 With child in the recovery position, clear mouth and nostrils of foreign material.

2 Tilt head back slightly.

3 Lift chin to bring tongue away from back of throat.

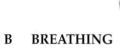
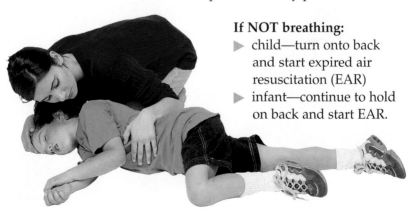

B   **BREATHING**

1 Look, listen and feel for breathing for up to 10 seconds.

2 **If breathing:**
  ▶ child—leave in recovery position
  ▶ infant—put in recovery position.

If NOT breathing:
  ▶ child—turn onto back and start expired air resuscitation (EAR)
  ▶ infant—continue to hold on back and start EAR.

EXPIRED AIR RESUSCITATION (EAR)

Note: Give up to 5 breaths to achieve at least 2 effective breaths.

INFANT (TO 1 YEAR)

1 Support the infant's head. Cover infant's mouth and nose with your mouth and give 2 gentle puffs of air from your cheeks, sufficient to make the infant's chest rise (2 effective breaths).

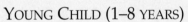

2 After the initial 2 puffs, check the pulse. If there is a pulse but no breathing, continue to inflate the lungs at a rate of 20 times per minute.

3 Check the pulse about every minute.

YOUNG CHILD (1–8 YEARS)

1 Hold child's nose and give 2 gentle breaths into the mouth sufficient to make the child's chest rise (2 effective breaths).

2 After the initial 2 breaths, check the pulse. If there is a pulse but no breathing, continue to inflate the lungs at a rate of 20 times per minute.

3 Check the pulse about every minute.

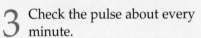

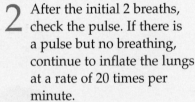

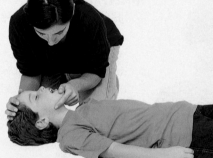

C CIRCULATION

If the child's heart has stopped beating or if you cannot feel a pulse, giving chest compressions will help maintain blood circulation through the heart and to the brain. **External chest compression (ECC) is always combined with EAR, the combination of techniques being known as cardiopulmonary resuscitation (CPR).**

Child (from 1 year): check carotid (neck) or radial (wrist) pulse, as for adults.

Infant: check brachial pulse—inner upper arm.

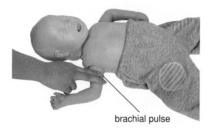

brachial pulse

Newborn: check apex beat—chest below left nipple.

Note: Check pulse for no more than 10 seconds before continuing resuscitation.

CARDIOPULMONARY RESUSCITATION (CPR)

Although CPR for young children and infants is similar to that used for adults and older children (over 8 years), there are some differences due to their smaller bodies and because respiratory arrest is more likely than cardiac arrest. Children have faster breathing rates, so the speed of your breaths must be adjusted. The pressure you give during compressions must also be adjusted.

Note: For a newborn baby (within minutes of birth) chest compressions should not be attempted by anyone untrained in neonatal resuscitation.

Give CPR

Give CPR (see steps at right); check pulse, then:

If the heartbeat returns, but there is no breathing

1 Continue EAR.

2 Seek help—take infant/child to the telephone with you if possible.

3 Check breathing and pulse about every minute.

If the child starts to breathe again

1 Place in recovery position.

2 Keep airway open.

3 Check vital signs closely until arrival of ambulance.

When to stop CPR

It is important to ensure that once CPR has commenced, there is no interruption, unless:
 ▶ the child shows signs of life
 ▶ qualified help arrives
 ▶ you are physically unable to continue

CARDIOPULMONARY RESUSCITATION (CPR)
INFANT (TO 1 YEAR)

1 Use 2 fingers (index and middle) over lower half of sternum to give chest compressions.

2 Compress chest approx. 1/3 depth of chest.

3 Give 5 chest compressions in 3 seconds followed by 1 breath (5:1).

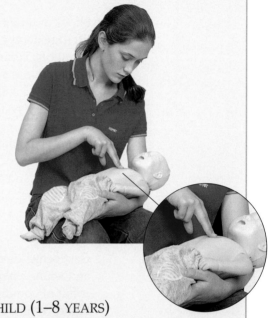

YOUNG CHILD (1–8 YEARS)

1 Use heel of one hand over lower half of sternum to give chest compressions.

2 Compress chest approx. 1/3 depth of chest.

3 Give 5 chest compressions in 3 seconds followed by 1 breath (5:1).

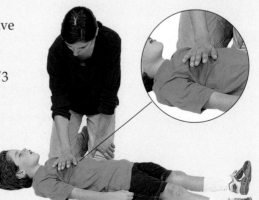

Note: Continue CPR for 1 minute then check pulse and breathing for no more than 10 seconds.

SHOCK

Shock in infants and children, as in adults, is a life-threatening condition that may occur as a result of a serious injury or illness, particularly when there is severe bleeding or fluid loss. It is a progressive condition involving the collapse of the circulatory system, and may lead to death.

Shock is not always readily apparent immediately after an injury. The signs and symptoms develop gradually and depend on the severity of the injury. Shock also depends on whether fluid loss continues and on the effectiveness of management of the injury.

Gastroenteritis can be particularly serious in infants and young children. If a child loses a lot of fluid as a result of vomiting or diarrhoea, there is a loss of blood volume which can mean there is insufficient blood to transport oxygen to the tissues. This leads to shock.

Signs and symptoms

▶ pale, cold and sweaty skin (often most notice-able on face, lips and under fingernails)
▶ shallow, fast breathing
▶ weak, rapid pulse

If there is severe shock, the casualty may also be restless, thirsty and nauseated, or may become drowsy, confused or unconscious. The casualty's extremities may turn bluish in colour.
TRY NOT to leave a child suffering from shock unattended—send someone else (if available) to phone for the ambulance.
DO NOT give the child anything to drink or eat—if thirsty, moisten lips with water.

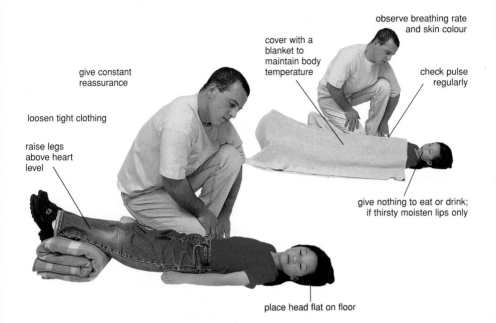

observe breathing rate and skin colour

cover with a blanket to maintain body temperature

give constant reassurance

check pulse regularly

loosen tight clothing

raise legs above heart level

give nothing to eat or drink; if thirsty moisten lips only

place head flat on floor

MANAGEMENT OF SHOCK

1 Follow DRABC and control severe bleeding.

DRABC ►

2 Reassure the casualty.

3 ☎ *Call 000 for an ambulance.*

4 Raise the casualty's legs above the level of the heart; place head flat on floor.

5 Dress any wounds or burns and immobilise any fractures.

6 Loosen any tight clothing at the neck, chest and waist.

7 Place a blanket or coat over casualty to maintain body temperature (**DO NOT** use a hot water bottle or other source of direct heat).

8 Monitor the casualty's breathing, pulse and skin colour at regular intervals.

9 **DO NOT** give anything to drink or eat—if casualty thirsty, moisten lips with water.

CHOKING

Infants and small children love to put things in their mouths. This can result in choking. Both toys and food may be responsible. Peanuts and hard sweets are especially dangerous for children under five.

Signs and symptoms   The child may be unable to breathe at all if the obstruction of the airway is complete. If the obstruction is partial, the child may be able to get some air in past the obstruction. Signs of a child choking include:

▶ having difficulty breathing
▶ trying to cry but making strange sounds or no sound at all
▶ making a whistling or 'crowing' noise
▶ turning blue in the face
▶ collapsing or being unconscious

MANAGEMENT OF CHOKING—INFANT (TO 1 YEAR)

Check airway and breathing to assess blockage

Partial blockage

1 Lie infant face down on your forearm with head low.

2 Support infant's head and shoulders on your hand.

3 Give 4 sharp slaps between shoulders.

4 Check in infant's mouth and remove any obstruction that may have come loose.

5 If blockage has not cleared:
☎ *call 000 for an ambulance.*

(continued next page)

58

Total blockage

1 Place infant face down on your lap.

2 Give 4 sharp slaps between shoulders.

3 Check for signs of breathing.

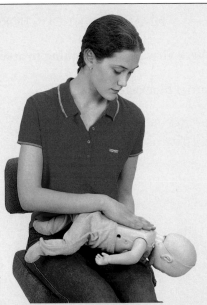

If still not breathing:

4 Give lateral chest thrusts by placing one hand on either side of the infant's chest below the armpits. Give up to 4 quick, squeezing thrusts on both sides simultaneously.

5 Check in infant's mouth and remove any obstruction that may have come loose; check for breathing.

6 If blockage has not cleared: ☎ *call 000 for an ambulance.*

7 Follow DRABC

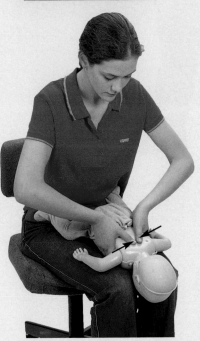

8 Repeat steps 4 and 5 until help arrives or blockage clears.

MANAGEMENT OF CHOKING—CHILD (1–8 YEARS)

Check airway and breathing to assess blockage

Partial blockage

1   Ask child to try to cough up obstruction.

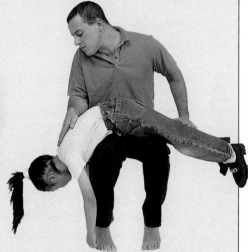

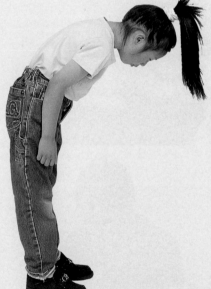

4   If blockage has not cleared:
     ☎ *call 000 for an ambulance.*

Total blockage

1   Place child face down on the floor or across your lap.

2   If unsuccessful, place child in position with head low and face down (up-end or bend over your knee).

2   Give 4 sharp blows between the shoulderblades.

3   Give 4 sharp blows between the shoulderblades.

3   Check for signs of breathing.

(continued next page)

If still not breathing:

4 Give lateral chest thrusts by placing one hand on either side of the child's chest below the armpits. Give up to 4 quick, squeezing thrusts on both sides simultaneously.

5 Check in mouth for any obstruction; check breathing.

6 If blockage has not cleared:
☎ *call 000 for an ambulance.*

7 Follow DRABC

8 Repeat steps 4 and 5 until help arrives or blockage clears.

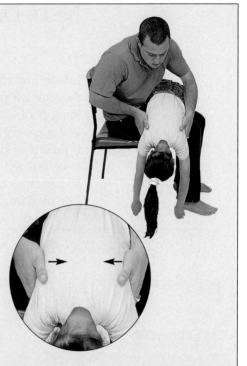

Preventing choking in infants

Food
- give small bite-sized pieces only, especially if infant has few teeth
- do not give peanuts, raisins, hard food etc.

Toys
- check toys regularly for loose parts and stitching tears
- check dummies for small parts or worn nipples—if worn, throw away
- do not let infants play with balloons
- keep all toys out of baby's bassinet

Preventing choking in children

Food
- supervise children when eating
- never give nuts to a child below school age
- insist that children sit still when eating
- grate apples and carrots for young children

Toys
- always supervise children playing with balloons—deflated balloons can cause choking
- check house for toys and other items that may cause choking—coins, pen tops, etc.

Near Drowning

Infants and children can drown very quickly if they are left unattended in a bath, near a swimming pool, at the beach or near a river or pond. Water is very attractive to young children. If infants or children fall into water, they have to be rescued quickly. There is a better than 50 per cent chance of saving an apparently drowned infant or child by giving resuscitation.

Management of Near Drowning

1   Assess the scene.

2   Lift casualty out of the water.

3   Carry casualty with the head lower than the chest.

4   Follow DRABC

5   Call an ambulance or take the casualty to hospital even if recovered.

6   Remove any wet clothing and cover casualty with a towel or blanket.

7   Monitor condition and resuscitate if necessary.

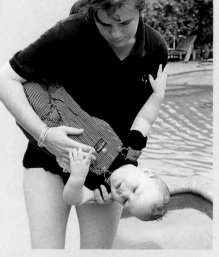

Water in the lungs and the effects of cold can increase resistance to EAR, so you may need to breathe more firmly and slowly to get the chest to rise.

8   Place in a recovery position if breathing.

Wound dressing and infection control

A first aid kit is a necessity for every first aider—indeed for every citizen. It contains the bandages, dressings, pads, gloves and other items needed to deal with any situation.

Knowing what each item is used for and how it is used is very important.

Sometimes first aiders will have to improvise because a first aid kit is not readily available. This chapter discusses the materials in your first aid kit and what materials can be used as substitutes.

Hygiene and awareness of infection transmission have high priority in first aid. Precautions to prevent infection and ways to minimise risk are discussed in this chapter.

WOUND DRESSING AND INFECTION CONTROL

All open wounds need some type of covering to help control bleeding, to prevent infection and to reduce pain. To do this, dressings and bandages are the main items used by the first aider. Different types of dressings and bandages are used, in varying ways, depending on the injury and on materials available.

Other items will also be used in dressing a wound—pads to help absorb blood or to give further protection, swabs for cleaning, tape to keep dressings in place, and a range of sundry items such as scissors and towels. These items are found in a Basic St John First Aid Kit. You can, of course, make up your own.

FIRST AID KIT

A first aid kit should be kept in your home, your car and in the workplace. The contents of first aid kits used in the workplace are covered by regulations in each State or Territory.

It is important to ensure that you regularly check the contents of your first aid kit to make sure they are clean, packets are properly sealed, expiry dates have not been exceeded, and that you have replaced any previously used items.

Although it is safer to use sterile bandages and dressings, there will be emergencies when you will not have a first aid kit immediately to hand. You will then have to use whatever materials you can find.

TIP

Check the contents of your first aid kit after every use.

Immediately replace any used and out-of-date items.

Contents of a
Basic St John
First Aid Kit

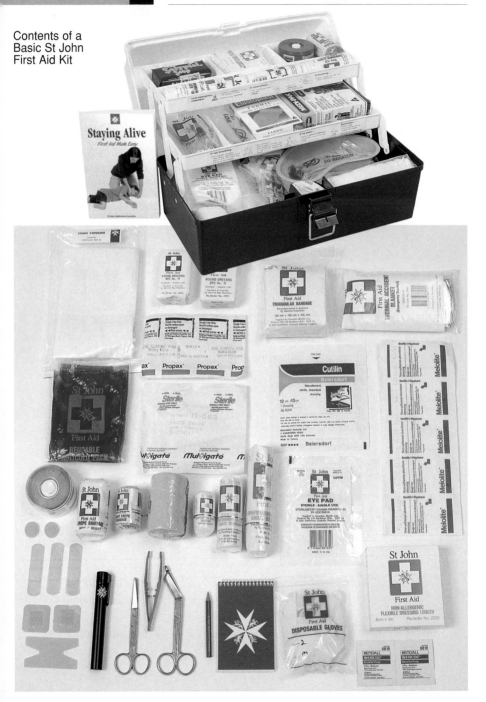

A BASIC ST JOHN FIRST AID KIT

ITEM	USE

Bandages

ITEM	USE
• two triangular bandages	• *for emergency dressings*
	• *as slings to support upper arm*
• two 10 cm crepe or conforming bandages	• *for pressure immobilisation after snakebite and some other bites and stings*
	• *to bind large/medium dressings in place*
• two 7.5 cm conforming bandages	• *to bind medium dressings in place*
• two 5 cm conforming bandages	• *to bind medium/small dressings in place*

Dressings

ITEM	USE
• two 10 cm x 10 cm non-adherent dressings	• *for use when you don't want the bandage to stick to the wound (e.g. burns, weeping or oozing wounds)*
• one no. 13 wound dressing	• *to control bleeding and protect moderate wounds*
• one no. 14 wound dressing	• *to control bleeding and protect major wounds*
• one no. 15 wound dressing	• *as an eye pad*
• one pkt of 25 adhesive shapes	• *for small cuts and abrasions*

Pads

ITEM	USE
• two 9 cm x 20 cm combine pads	• *for padding of major injuries*
	• *for placing over non-adherent dressings*
• four eye pads	• *for covering wounded eyes*

ITEM	USE

Swabs
- nine 7.5 cm x 7.5 cm x 3 cm gauze swabs
- six alcohol swabs

- *for cleaning wounds and surrounding areas*
- *for cleaning first aider's hands*

Other
- one roll of adhesive tape (at least 24 mm wide and 2.5 m long)
- three disposable hand towels

- one pair of stainless steel scissors

- three 30 ml saline eyewash

- six safety pins
- Stingose™ gel

- three medium plastic bags

- one pair of stainless steel tweezers
- one thermo blanket

- note pad and pencil
- four pairs of disposable gloves

- *to secure light dressings*

- *for general cleaning (not wounds)*
- *to cut dressings, bandages etc. and to cut away clothing*
- *for eye irrigation and wound cleaning*
- *to secure bandages and slings*
- *to soothe irritation of insect bites and stings*
- *various uses e.g. to make icepacks, carry water, seal an open chest wound, store dressings*
- *for removing splinters etc.*
- *for protection against the elements, to prevent loss of body heat*
- *for recording times and details*
- *to assist in preventing cross infection*

THE SKIN

The skin plays an important role in protecting the body from infection. It also performs a number of other important functions. The skin:

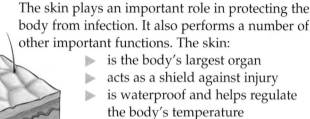

▶ is the body's largest organ
▶ acts as a shield against injury
▶ is waterproof and helps regulate the body's temperature
▶ alerts the brain to changes in the environment

epidermis

dermis

deep fascia

sweat gland

hair follicle

nerve

subcutaneous fat

The outer layer or epidermis acts as a barrier to bacteria and other organisms that cause infection. A deeper layer, called the dermis, contains the main nerve structures, sweat and oil glands and blood vessels. There is an abundance of nerves in the skin which are sensitive to touch, heat, cold and pain, and which transmit these sensations to the brain.

Because the skin has a plentiful supply of nerves and blood vessels, most superficial injuries are likely to bleed and be painful. When an injury causes a break in the outer layer of skin, there is the potential for germs to enter and cause infection. Any wound can become infected if it is not properly cared for.

MINIMISE INFECTION BY:

▶ washing and drying your hands thoroughly before and after management
▶ wearing clean disposable gloves
▶ avoiding coughing, sneezing

or talking while managing the wound
▶ handling the wound only when it is necessary to control severe bleeding
▶ using sterile or clean dressings

Types of Wounds

Wounds are classified according to the type of damage they cause to the skin and tissues under the skin. A wound can be open or closed.

OPEN WOUNDS

An open wound is where there is a break in the outer layer of skin. Open wounds may be minor (e.g. a surface scrape) or more severe (e.g. when an object penetrates deeply to underlying layers). Although the amount of bleeding will depend on how bad the injury is, any open wound provides a gateway for germs to enter the body and cause infection.

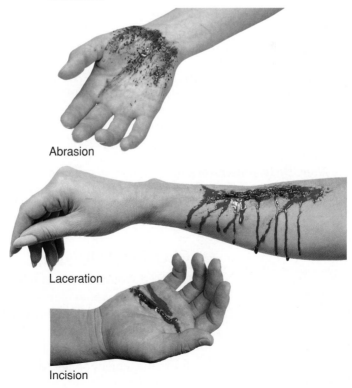

Abrasion

Laceration

Incision

When you are caring for an open wound, you have to decide if the wound is major or not. If damage to the skin is superficial and/or bleeding is minimal, the wound can be considered minor. All other wounds should be considered major wounds and treated as such.

MANAGEMENT OF OPEN WOUNDS

Minor wounds

1 Clean the wound thoroughly with gauze soaked in sterile or cooled boiled water, or under running tap-water.

2 Apply a non-stick dressing.

Major wounds

1 Follow DRABC.

2 Control bleeding.

3 Clean the wound as well as possible.

4 Apply a sterile or clean dressing.

5 Seek medical aid.

Note: Dirty, penetrating, or open wounds should be examined by a doctor, as tetanus or other serious infections may result.

CLOSED WOUNDS

A closed wound is one in which there is no break in the outer layer of skin, so any damage and bleeding will be internal (e.g. a bruise or contusion). As the outer layer of skin is left intact, there is not the same risk of infection. (See chapter five for management of closed wounds.)

WOUND DRESSING

The main aims of wound dressing are to:
▶ control bleeding
▶ protect the wound from possible infection

Your basic first aid kit contains all the materials you need for this, whatever the severity and type of injury. The way in which you use and apply these materials will vary with the type of injury and where the injury is located on the body. There may, however, be times when you either do not have a first aid kit nearby or your kit is incomplete. Then you will need to improvise.

DRESSINGS

Dressings are placed directly on a wound to:
▶ absorb blood and other body fluids
▶ keep the wound clean
▶ help protect the wound from infection
▶ reduce pain

General principles for applying dressings

▶ wash hands before pulling on clean disposable gloves
▶ use a sterile dressing that extends about 2 cms past the edges of the wound
▶ do not touch the surface that will contact the wound
▶ if the wound is minor, clean with sterile or clean water before applying the dressing
▶ replace at least once a day any dressing which becomes wet or soiled
▶ wash hands after removing gloves

Adhesive dressings

Adhesive dressings are generally used for minor wounds. They have an absorbent pad attached to an adhesive strip or backing. They come in many shapes and sizes and may be packaged individually within packets or be available as a continuous strip.

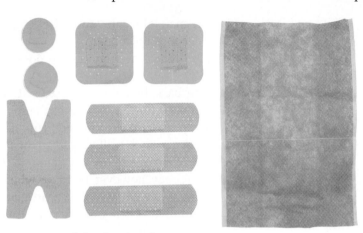

Adhesive dressings

Non-adherent dressings

Non-adherent dressings can be used with any injury, but are especially useful for burns and abrasions where the injury is to the surface of the skin and it is important to prevent blood and fluids sticking to the dressing. Because they are not adherent, they can usually be removed easily.

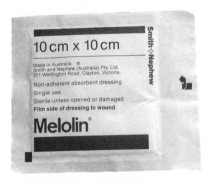

Non-adherent dressings

Combine and BPC dressings

Combine and BPC dressings combine a bandage and pad-dressing in one unit and are used for large or deep wounds. Because they are made of layers of gauze and cotton wool, their bulk is useful for controlling bleeding and for absorbing discharge.

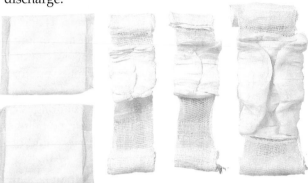

Combine and BPC dressings

To apply a combine or BPC dressing:

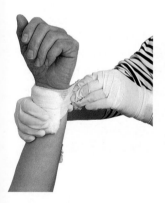

1 Hold an end of bandage in each hand and position pad on wound.

2 Wrap shorter end around limb or trunk of body to hold in place.

3 Wrap longer end over dressing until covered.

4 Tie ends with a reef knot.

Adhesive dressings	Non-adherent dressings	Combine and BPC dressings
• for minor wounds • come in many shapes and sizes	• for any wound • most useful for skin surface injuries (e.g. burns, abrasions)	• for large/very large or deep wounds • used when bulk is needed to control bleeding or absorb discharge in a large area

BANDAGES

A **bandage** is any material used to wrap or cover a wound. Bandages are used to:

- keep dressings in place
- control bleeding
- protect a wound from dirt and infection
- give support and pain relief
- restrict movement
- minimise swelling
- immobilise fractures (usually with splints)

Triangular bandages

Triangular bandages can be used as dressings, pads, padding or slings. If used to bandage a wound, they should be secured with a reef knot. They can be made by cutting a one metre square piece of cloth diagonally into two triangular pieces. If the triangular bandage is too large for your needs, fold it in half.

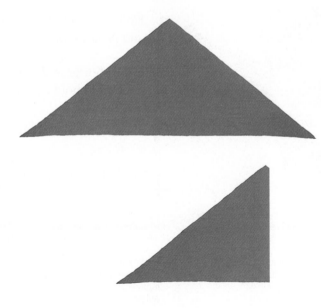

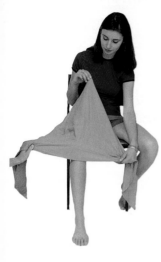

Triangular bandages can be used to secure a dressing or padding at the knee or elbow when a roller bandage is not available.

1 Fold a narrow hem across base of bandage.

2 Place the centre of base on leg below kneecap with the point towards top of leg.

3 Take bandage ends around leg, cross over at back and bring to front.

4 Tie above kneecap using a reef knot.

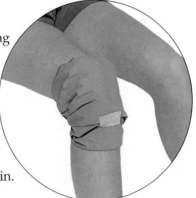

5 Fold the rest of bandage down and secure with tape or tuck in.

While a triangular bandage can be used to hold a dressing on the head in place, or to bandage a foot or hand, these tasks can be more easily accomplished using an elastic (conforming) roller bandage.

Roller bandages

Roller bandages can be elastic (conforming) or non-elastic. They are made from long strips of material—cotton, gauze, elastic or synthetic—and come in varying widths. They can be used to wrap around parts of the body that are fairly straight, such as the wrist or fingers, to apply pressure to control bleeding, to keep dressings in place and to support an injured part.

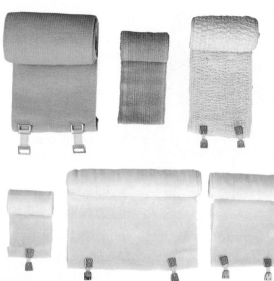

Roller bandages

To apply a roller bandage:

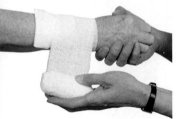

1 Place 'tail' end of bandage below the wound, keeping roll of bandage uppermost.

2 Make one full turn over limb to hold 'tail' in place.

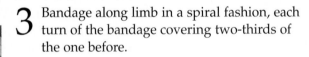

3 Bandage along limb in a spiral fashion, each turn of the bandage covering two-thirds of the one before.

OR

Bandage along limb using a figure of eight pattern.

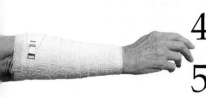

4 Fasten the end with adhesive tape, use clip provided, or tuck in.

5 Check circulation and adjust bandage if necessary (see p. 79).

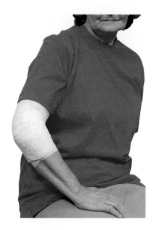

Roller bandages can be used to bandage the elbow, knee, hand or foot. When applying a roller bandage to the elbow or knee, make alternate turns above and below the joint (figure of eight pattern).

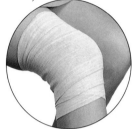

To apply a roller bandage to the hand or foot:

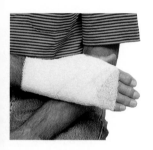

1   Secure the 'tail' of bandage with one turn around wrist or ankle.

2   Bring the next turn in a diagonal from wrist or ankle to little finger or toe.

3   Take bandage across palm of hand or sole of foot and back to wrist or ankle.

4   Continue to use a figure of eight pattern to cover hand or foot (leave fingers or toes exposed).

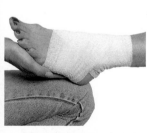

5   Make final turn around wrist or ankle and secure with adhesive tape or tuck in.

6   Check circulation to ensure bandage is not too tight (see p. 79).

Elastic roller bandages are usually used for sprains and other musculoskeletal injuries where an even pressure is necessary to support the joint or to reduce or prevent swelling.

**Tubular gauze
bandages**

Tubular gauze bandages are made of seamless stretch gauze tubing and are used to bandage fingers and toes. Tubular bandages are applied with a specially designed applicator or are stretched by hand to cover and retain a dressing. To apply:

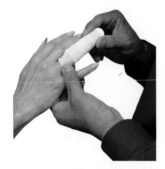

1 Cut a piece of bandage approximately three times as long as finger to be bandaged.

2 Push all of gauze tube over the applicator.

3 Push applicator over the finger.

4 Hold end of tubular bandage at base of finger.

5 Pull applicator off finger.

6 Rotate applicator once or twice to twist gauze bandage at end of finger.

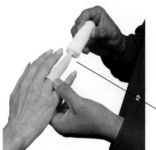

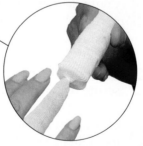

7 Push applicator over finger to apply second layer of bandage.

8 Secure end with tape.

CHECKING CIRCULATION

Circulation in the hand or foot must be checked regularly after any bandage, splint or sling has been applied. This is important as swelling of the limb can make the bandage tighter. If circulation is impaired the bandage must be loosened.

Signs and symptoms of a bandage being too tight

▶ absent pulse below the bandage
▶ swelling
▶ paleness, blueness or coldness of the fingers or toes
▶ numbness and tingling (pins and needles) of the fingers or toes
▶ pain

How to check circulation

▶ check skin colour—if not normal, circulation could be impaired
▶ check skin temperature—if cold, circulation could be impaired
▶ check for circulation in fingers or toes: press fingernail or toenail until it turns white, then release—if colour returns within 2 seconds, blood flow is unrestricted

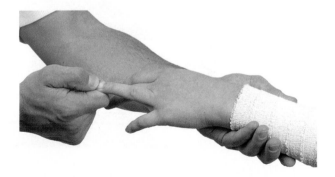

PADS

Pads are thick and bulky and are used to:
- help control bleeding
- absorb blood and other secretions
- help prevent infection
- protect sensitive areas
- give extra padding

Triangular bandages can be folded and used as a pad. To do this:

1   Place point of triangle down on base.

2   Fold in half to make a broad bandage.

3   Fold in half again to make a narrow bandage.

4 Bring ends to middle (do twice).

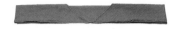

5 Fold in half again to make a pad.

(Bandages can be folded this way for storage.)

BANDAGES	DRESSINGS	PADS

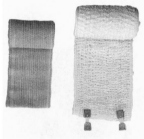 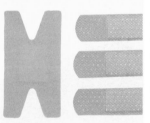 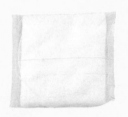

Used to:	**Used to:**	**Used to:**
• apply direct pressure to control bleeding	• control bleeding	• help control bleeding
• keep dressings and splints in position	• prevent infection	• help prevent infection
• give support and relief from pain	• protect wounds	• protect sensitive areas (e.g. eye)
• restrict movement	• ease pain	• give extra padding
• immobilise fractures	**They should be:**	**They should be:**
• minimise swelling	• sterile or clean	• clean
• protect from dirt and infection	• non-adherent	
They should be:		
• sterile or clean		

SPLINTS

Splints are used to immobilise and support a limb or injured part of the body. This is particularly important if the casualty has to be moved.

Although commercial splints are available, splints can be improvised using any item or material that is suitable. Padded boards, tree limbs, rolled newspapers or a length of wood can each be used as a splint. An injured leg can even be splinted to the uninjured leg. In fact, any material which is the required length and wide enough to support the injured body part can be used as a splint.

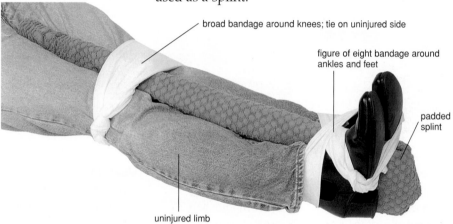

broad bandage around knees; tie on uninjured side

figure of eight bandage around ankles and feet

padded splint

uninjured limb

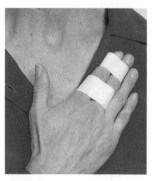

The splint has to be long enough to extend past the injured area to ensure the limb or entire body part is immobilised. Padding is usually placed between the splint and the natural curves of the limb such as at the elbow, knee, wrist and ankle, or where points of pressure may occur.

A broken finger or toe can best be splinted by placing gauze between it and the adjoining digit and taping them together.

SLINGS

The collar and cuff sling

The collar and cuff sling is a useful sling for a fracture of the upper arm or an injured hand.

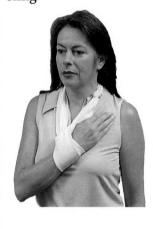

1 Make a clove hitch, using a narrow bandage.

2 Put the loops over the wrist of the injured arm.

3 Gently elevate the injured arm against the casualty's chest.

4 Tie bandage ends together around neck using reef knot positioned in hollow of collarbone.

The St John sling

The St John sling supports the elbow and prevents arm from pulling on an injured shoulder or collarbone.

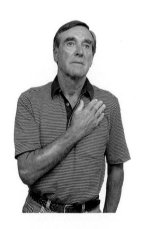

1 Place casualty's arm naturally by the side with elbow bent (if able) and forearm across chest (fingers point to opposite shoulder).

2 Drape an open triangular bandage over forearm, with point past elbow and one end over uninjured shoulder.

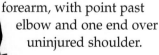

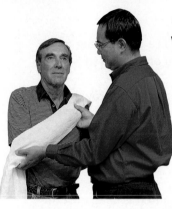

3 Supporting the arm, tuck the base (long side) of bandage under hand and forearm and around elbow.

4 Bring the lower end up diagonally across casualty's back to meet other end at shoulder.

5 Gently adjust height of sling.

6 Tie ends as close to fingers as possible.

7 Tuck the point firmly in between forearm and bandage to support elbow.

8 When you are sure sling is firm, secure the fold with a safety pin.

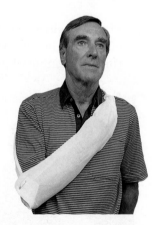

9 Check the circulation by applying gentle pressure to a fingernail (normal colour should return rapidly to the nail when you stop pressing it).

The full arm sling

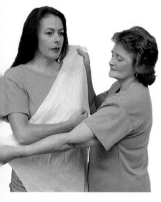

The full arm sling is used to support an injured forearm and/or wrist.

1 Place an open triangular bandage between chest and injured arm, with one end of the base length over uninjured shoulder and the other end pointing towards the ground (point of bandage is near elbow).

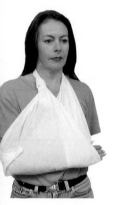

2 Bring the injured forearm slightly above the horizontal position.

3 Tie lower end of bandage to upper end in the hollow above collarbone on injured side (use a reef knot).

4 Carefully arrange bandage so the fingers are showing.

5 Bring the point of bandage to the front of elbow of injured arm and secure with a safety pin.

6 Check the circulation by applying gentle pressure to a fingernail (normal colour should return rapidly to the nail when you stop pressing it).

Improvised slings

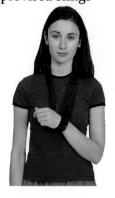

If there is no bandage available to make a sling, the casualty's clothing can be used to provide support. You can turn up the bottom of a jacket or shirt, use a belt or a tie, or place the hand inside a partially buttoned up shirt or jacket.

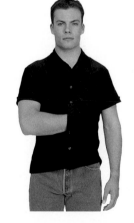

KNOTS

The reef knot is used to tie bandages because it does not slip, can be untied quite easily, lies flat and does not dig into the wound.

1 Take an end of the bandage in each hand.

2 Place the right-hand end over the left-hand end.

3 Turn it under and bring to the top so that it is now on the left.

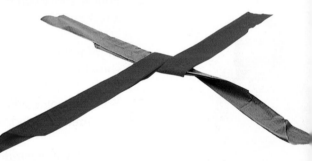

4 Place the new left-hand end over the new right-hand end.

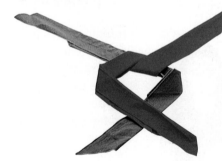

5 Turn it under and bring to the top so that it is now on the right.

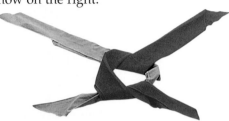

6 Tighten by pulling evenly on both ends.

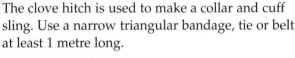

The clove hitch

The clove hitch is used to make a collar and cuff sling. Use a narrow triangular bandage, tie or belt at least 1 metre long.

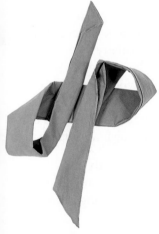

1 Make two loops (the ends go in opposite directions).

2 Place your hands under the loops and bring them together.

3 Slide the loops over casualty's arm and position them at wrist.

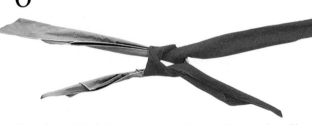

4 Tie the ends around neck (reef knot in hollow of collarbone).

HYGIENE AND COMMUNICABLE DISEASES

HYGIENE

Ensuring cleanliness at the site of an accident is extremely important. Unless the first aider takes all necessary precautions, wounds can become infected and this may lengthen recovery. It is also possible that infection could be passed on to the first aider. Therefore it is important to assume that every situation is potentially infectious.

Hygiene before and during first aid

▶ treat all people equally—assume all are infectious
▶ wash hands thoroughly with soap and water before first aid; dry thoroughly
▶ clean hands with hand wipes or medi-preps if soap and water not available
▶ wash hands after dressing an open wound
▶ wear disposable gloves whenever possible
▶ change gloves for each casualty
▶ change gloves if torn when giving first aid
▶ avoid touching an open wound
▶ cover any exposed wounds with a dressing
▶ do not touch infected wounds or potentially infected material (e.g. dressings) with bare hands

Hygiene after first aid

▶ **wash and dry hands thoroughly**
▶ **soak clothing** in cold water for at least 60 minutes then machine-wash using hot water and detergent
▶ **clean contaminated surfaces**—cover for 30 minutes with paper towels which have been soaked in the strongest recommended bleach solution
Note: Use bleach only in well-ventilated areas.

▶ **burn combustible waste materials**
▶ **place non-combustible waste materials**
inside two plastic bags, tie securely and
dispose of safely; DO NOT put in rubbish
bin—seek expert advice from your local
hospital or doctor
▶ **wash and disinfect resuscitation mask—**
wash in warm soapy water and soak in a 10%
solution of pure bleach for not less than 10
minutes. Rinse in plain cold water and air dry
in a clean environment
*Note: Valves and filters in pocket masks are
'single use only' and cannot be disinfected.*

Remember

▶ if you are splashed with blood or bodily
fluids or come into contact with them, wash
thoroughly with soap and water
▶ if your lips, mouth, tongue, eyes or broken
skin come into contact with blood or bodily
fluids, wash thoroughly
▶ if your skin is punctured by a sharp object
that may be contaminated, wash thoroughly
with soap and running water
*Note: If any of the above occur seek medical
advice promptly.*

St John Ambulance Australia has prepared a
Communicable Diseases Protection Pack to be
used in conjunction with first aid kits. It contains
a face mask, disposable goggles and gloves.

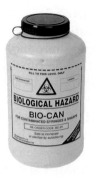

Container for used sharps (e.g. syringe, blood-testing needle)

COMMUNICABLE DISEASES

The first aider should remain aware that some illnesses can be transmitted from person to person when giving first aid. Although rare, this may happen if there is direct contact between one person's blood, other bodily fluids, or infectious areas, and another person's mucous membranes or broken skin (cuts, grazes or scratches).

Such illnesses include colds, influenza, measles, mumps, glandular fever, hepatitis, human immunodeficiency virus (HIV), acquired immune deficiency syndrome (AIDS), herpes, tuberculosis (TB), some forms of meningitis and some skin infections (such as cold sores).

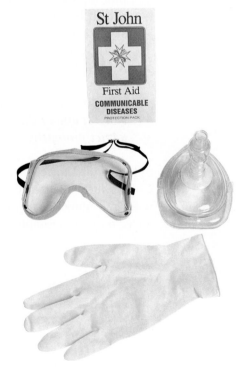

Communicable Diseases Protection Pack

In the first aid situation, these diseases may be passed on by:

- blood and bodily fluids (e.g. saliva, vomit, pus, urine, faeces)
- infected hypodermic needles or sharp objects
- droplets (e.g. nasal, throat, or airway secretions)

First aiders should protect both themselves and the casualty by using disposable gloves, eye protection, face masks and protective clothing as appropriate.

How to Remove Gloves *

Once gloves are used in first aid, they are contaminated and can be a source of infection. They must be taken off without touching the outside surface and, where possible, hands washed and dried immediately.

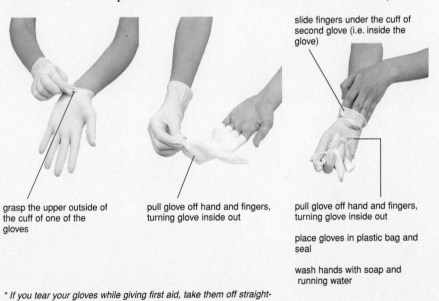

slide fingers under the cuff of second glove (i.e. inside the glove)

grasp the upper outside of the cuff of one of the gloves

pull glove off hand and fingers, turning glove inside out

pull glove off hand and fingers, turning glove inside out

place gloves in plastic bag and seal

wash hands with soap and running water

If you tear your gloves while giving first aid, take them off straight-away. Wash and dry your hands and put on a new pair of gloves.

Chapter

5

Wounds and bleeding

Blood is vital for the body to function properly. Blood has many important functions—transporting oxygen and nutrients to all parts of the body, eliminating wastes, transporting antibodies to protect against disease and germs, and maintaining a constant body temperature.

When there is an open wound and blood loss, how should the first aider respond? Bleeding must be stopped and the wound must be protected. The possibility of infection and shock has to be considered whether the wound is major or minor, and whether or not there is major blood loss.

Internal bleeding poses special challenges to the first aider. It has to be recognised and treated with care. It can be difficult to assess how serious internal bleeding is. What are the signs of internal bleeding? How do you manage internal bleeding?

Some wounds are life-threatening and need urgent attention. Others may be minor but can still cause pain and, if not managed correctly, become more serious later. This chapter looks at a number of wound types and how to manage them.

BLEEDING

Bleeding is the loss of blood from the blood vessels. This can be external and obvious, or internal (within the body) where it often cannot be seen. Severe or continued bleeding may lead to collapse and death, so the first aider must develop skills to control severe bleeding.

Bleeding is classified according to the type of blood vessel—artery, vein or capillary—that is damaged.

Arterial blood is oxygen-rich, bright red in colour and under pressure, so it spurts from the wound. Because this makes it more difficult for the blood to clot, arterial bleeding is hardest to control.

Venous blood (from the veins) is oxygen-depleted, dark red in colour and under less pressure. It flows from a wound more evenly and without spurting.

Capillary bleeding is the most common form of bleeding and is usually slow because the blood vessels are small and under low pressure. Clotting occurs easily with this type of bleeding. If capillaries are ruptured beneath the skin's surface, blood escapes into the surrounding tissues and bruising results.

Whether the bleeding is external and therefore obvious, or internal and not obvious, it is important for the first aider to know from other signs and symptoms how serious the blood loss is.

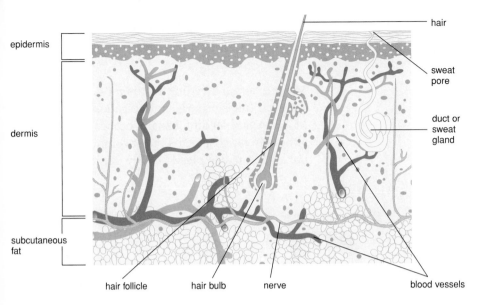

epidermis

dermis

subcutaneous
fat

hair follicle   hair bulb   nerve

hair

sweat
pore

duct or
sweat
gland

blood vessels

**Signs and symptoms
of major bleeding**

- faintness or dizziness
- restlessness
- nausea
- thirst
- weak, rapid pulse
- cold, clammy skin
- rapid, gasping breathing
- pallor
- sweating
- progressive loss of consciousness (drowsy,
  irrational or unconscious)

External Bleeding

Major external bleeding occurs most often after a deep cut (incision) or tear (laceration) in the skin. Most severe bleeding usually occurs from arteries, although varicose veins (most commonly found in the legs) can also bleed heavily *(see p. 113)*.

TYPES OF WOUNDS

	Bruise (Contusion)	Abrasion	Cut (Incision)
Kind of wound	closed	open	open
Caused by	blow from something blunt	skin being scraped across a hard surface	something sharp (e.g. knife or glass)
Injury causes	vessels under skin to bleed into surrounding tissues	outer layer of skin and tiny underlying blood vessels to be exposed	skin, soft tissue or muscles to be severed
Management	• RICE *(see p. 122)*	• cleanse wound • apply non-adherent dressing	• cleanse wound thoroughly with sterile gauze soaked in sterile water or cooled, boiled water • apply non-adherent dressing

The first aider should attempt to assess the amount of blood lost from a wound. The total quantity of blood in the human body varies according to size. An adult can lose 500 ml of blood without any harm, but in an infant the loss of 300 ml might cause death.

TYPES OF WOUNDS

	Laceration	**Puncture**	**Tear (Avulsion)**
Kind of wound	open	open	open
Caused by	machinery, barbed wire, teeth or claws	blunt or pointed instruments	something sharp (e.g. a knife)
Injury causes	skin and underlying tissue damage	skin and underlying tissue and sometimes internal organ damage	skin and other soft tissues to be partially or completely torn away
Management	• cleanse wound thoroughly with sterile gauze soaked in sterile water or cooled, boiled water • apply non-adherent dressing	• cleanse wound thoroughly with sterile gauze soaked in sterile water or cooled, boiled water • apply non-adherent dressing	• return skin to original position if possible • apply pressure to wound using a dressing and a pad to control any bleeding • bandage

Aims in managing bleeding

Ensure your hands are clean and gloved— if possible.

▶ control bleeding
- apply pressure to the wound to restrict the flow of blood and allow normal clotting to occur (use a dressing and a pad)
- raise the injured part to slow the flow of blood and encourage clotting
- maintain pressure on the pad (use a narrow folded triangular bandage or roller bandage)

▶ minimise shock—this may result from extensive loss of blood or emotional distress

▶ minimise the risk of infection—cover wound with a sterile bandage

▶ get medical aid

Major external bleeding requires rapid medical attention. However, where there is extensive blood loss, it can distract from the priorities of resuscitation. Rarely is blood loss so great that the heart stops.

If severe bleeding from a limb cannot be controlled by direct pressure, it may be necessary to apply pressure to the pressure points. These are found on the main artery above the wound. When bleeding has been controlled, remove pressure on the pressure point and reapply direct pressure to the wound. If a cut artery is spurting, it may be necessary to pinch the cut artery between finger and thumb. Severe bleeding is serious and the extent of bleeding may be hidden. It is therefore important to **act quickly!**

Pressure points

MANAGEMENT OF EXTERNAL BLEEDING

1 Follow DRABC.

DRABC

2 Lie casualty down if bleeding is severe.

3 Remove or cut clothing to expose the wound.

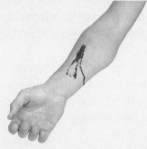

4 Apply direct pressure to the wound using a dressing and a pad (use gloves if available).

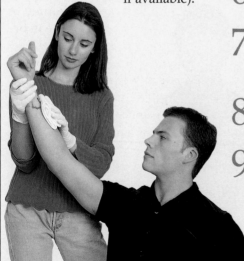

5 Bandage pad in place.

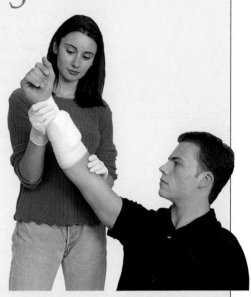

6 Raise and rest the injured part when possible.

7 If bleeding continues, place another pad on top and firmly bandage in place.

8 Give nothing by mouth.

9 ☎ *Call 000 for an ambulance.* if bleeding is severe or persistent.

WHEN TO USE A CONSTRICTIVE BANDAGE

Occasionally, in major limb injuries such as partial amputations or shark attack, severe bleeding cannot be controlled by direct pressure. In this sort of situation only, it may be necessary to resort to the application of a constrictive bandage above the elbow or knee to restrict arterial blood flow. But great care must be taken as its prolonged use can lead to tissues being starved of blood and dying.

The constrictive bandage

1 Use a firm cloth, at least 7.5 cms wide and about 75 cms long (improvise from clothing or by using a folded triangular bandage).

2 Bind the cloth strip firmly around the injured limb—between elbow and shoulder, or knee and pelvis—until a pulse can no longer be felt beyond the constrictive bandage and bleeding has been controlled.

3 Note the time of application; write this on the casualty in pen or lipstick.

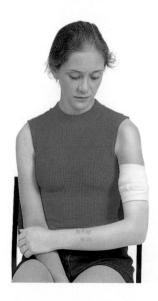

4 ☎ *Call 000 for an ambulance.*

5 After 30 minutes, release the bandage and check for bleeding:

> ▶ **if there is no bleeding**, remove the bandage
> ▶ **if bleeding recommences**, apply direct pressure
> ▶ **if this is unsuccessful**, reapply the constrictive bandage and recheck every 30 minutes.

Ensure bandage is clearly visible and a written tag is on the casualty. Inform medical aid of the position of bandage and time of application.

Note: In the rare cases where an (arterial) constrictive bandage is required, if it is applied too loosely, the bleeding can be made worse. It must stop the arterial pulse.

Major Wounds

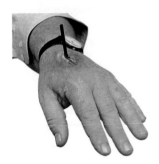

EMBEDDED OBJECT

When a foreign object such as a knife or branch is embedded in the wound and has penetrated into tissue, **DO NOT** try to remove it.

DO NOT exert any pressure over the object. **DO NOT** try to cut the end of the object unless its size makes it unmanageable. The object may be plugging the wound and restricting bleeding. Removing it may result in severe bleeding or may damage deep structures.

Management of Embedded Object

1. Control bleeding by applying pressure to the surrounding areas but not on the foreign object.

2. Place padding around the object or place a ring pad over the object and a bandage over the padding.

3. If the length of the object is such that it is protruding outside the pad, take care to bandage only each side of the object.

4. ☎ *Call 000 for an ambulance.*

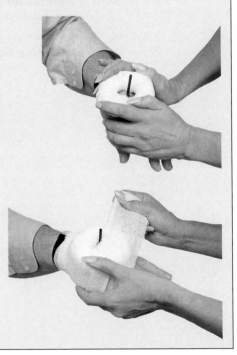

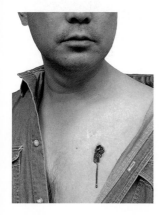

PENETRATING WOUNDS

Penetrating wounds are serious and may occur when a knife or high velocity object (e.g. a bullet) has penetrated the skin. The penetration may be deep and infection may occur. There may also be a second wound where the object has left the body and this must also be treated.

MANAGEMENT OF PENETRATING WOUNDS

1 Control bleeding—apply direct pressure around the wound.

2 Keep wound as clean as possible.

3 Cut away or remove clothing covering the wound.

4 If wound not bleeding, carefully clean out loose dirt.

5 **DO NOT** try to pick out foreign material embedded in the wound.

6 Apply a sterile or clean dressing.

7 Rest the injured part in a comfortable position.

8 ☎ *Call 000 for an ambulance.*

ABDOMINAL INJURIES

Abdominal injuries are dealt with in detail in chapter seven, Chest and Abdominal Injuries *(see p. 150).*

BLAST INJURIES

Blast injuries can result from an explosion in the workplace (e.g. from explosives or chemicals) or at home (e.g. from a gas heater). The casualty may be injured because of being thrown by the blast, struck by material thrown by the blast, or may suffer injuries to the lungs, stomach or intestines caused by shock waves from the blast.

Signs and symptoms include

▶ coughing up frothy blood
▶ chest pain
▶ possible bleeding from ears
▶ possible fractures
▶ multiple soft tissue injuries
▶ shock

MANAGEMENT OF BLAST INJURIES

1 Follow DRABC. **DRABC**

5 Care for wounds and burns.

2 ☎ *Call 000 for an ambulance.*

6 Immobilise any fractures.

3 Place casualty in comfortable position.

7 Monitor breathing and other vital signs.

4 Control bleeding.

AMPUTATED PARTS

An amputation occurs when a part of the body such as a toe, finger or leg is partly or completely cut off, or is torn off. The first aider aims to:

▶ minimise blood loss and shock
▶ preserve the amputated part

Because it may be possible to re-attach a finger or limb by microsurgery, the first aider will need to care for the amputated part in addition to the casualty.

MANAGEMENT OF AMPUTATIONS

The casualty

1 Follow DRABC.

2 Apply direct pressure to the wound and raise the limb to control blood loss.

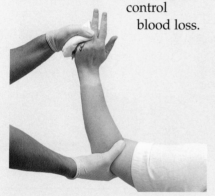

3 Apply a sterile dressing and bandage.

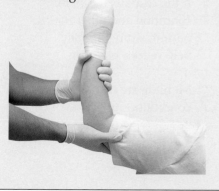

The amputated part

1 **DO NOT** wash or soak the amputated part in water or any other liquid.

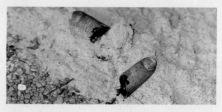

2 Wrap the part in gauze or material and place in a water-tight container, such as a sealed plastic bag.

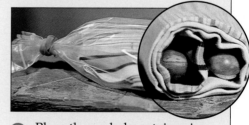

3 Place the sealed container in cold water which has had ice added to it—the severed part should not be in direct contact with ice.

4 Send to hospital with the casualty.

WOUNDS TO HEAD AND FACE

BLEEDING FROM THE SCALP

The head is easily injured because it lacks the padding of other parts of the body. An injury to this part of the body is of particular concern because of the possibility of injury to the skull.

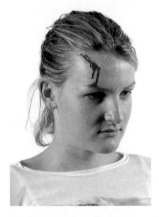 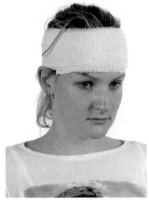

MANAGEMENT OF BLEEDING FROM THE SCALP

1 Follow DRABC.

2 **If you suspect a fracture** control bleeding with gentle pressure around the wound.

3 **If there appears to be no fracture** control bleeding with firm, direct pressure (wear gloves; use a pad if available).

4 If the casualty's general condition and other injuries permit, sitting up may help reduce bleeding.

5 Monitor the casualty's condition.

EAR WOUNDS

Ear injuries are common. Sport injuries and falls can damage the outer soft tissue. Bleeding can be controlled by applying pressure to affected area.

A direct blow to the head or pushing something into the ear may result in internal injury to the eardrum. Foreign objects—beads, stones, grass seeds—can become lodged in the canal. These can sometimes be removed by tilting head to side, pulling down on earlobe and gently shaking head.

DO NOT put anything in ear to try to remove object.

MANAGEMENT OF EAR WOUNDS

Bleeding from within the ear

1 Follow DRABC. **DRABC**

2 **DO NOT** plug ear canal.

3 **DO NOT** administer drops of any kind.

4 Allow fluid to drain freely.

5 Place casualty on side with affected ear down.

6 Place a sterile pad between ear and the ground.

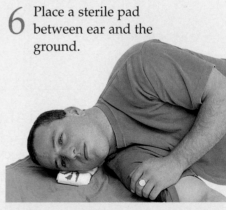

7 ☎ *Call 000 for an ambulance.*

MANAGEMENT OF EAR WOUNDS

Foreign object in ear

1 Look in the ear to identify the object and to see how deeply it is lodged.

2 **DO NOT** attempt to remove object.

3 Seek medical aid.

Small insect in ear

1 Gently pour some vegetable oil (water if oil not available), warmed to body temperature, in the ear.

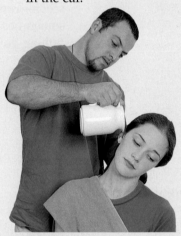

2 If insect does not float out, seek medical aid.

DENTAL INJURIES AND WOUNDS

Bleeding may result from a blow to the mouth which knocks teeth out, a tooth extraction or a loose tooth. The most important action is to ensure the casualty maintains a clear airway.

If a tooth is knocked out, save it. If you can, gently replace it. If you are unable to place it back in its socket, clean the tooth and store it in the casualty's saliva or in milk until dental attention is available.

To replace a knocked out tooth for a conscious and cooperative casualty

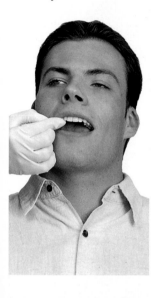

1   Gently clean dirt off tooth with casualty's own saliva or milk or if not available, use sterile saline solution.

2   Put tooth back in open socket.

3   Ask casualty to hold tooth in place. If unable to replant, wrap tooth in plastic or store in milk or sterile saline and rush casualty and tooth to a dentist.

4   **If tooth has been in contact with dirt or soil**, advise having a tetanus injection.

5   Advise seeing a dentist as soon as possible.

MANAGEMENT OF DENTAL INJURIES AND WOUNDS

1   Maintain a clear airway.

2   Ensure tongue is clear of tooth socket.

3   Place firm pad of gauze over socket.

4   Instruct casualty to bite firmly on gauze.

5   If bleeding continues, seek medical or dental aid.

NOSEBLEEDS

Nosebleeds can have various causes such as a blow to the nose, excessive blowing, sneezing, high blood pressure and changes in altitude. Many nosebleeds have no obvious cause.

MANAGEMENT OF NOSEBLEEDS

1   Ask casualty to breathe through mouth and not to blow nose.

2   Sit casualty up, head slightly forward.

3   Apply finger and thumb pressure on soft part of nostrils below bridge of nose for at least 10 minutes.

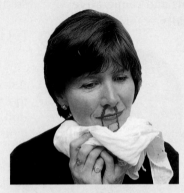

4   Loosen tight clothing around neck.

5   Place cold wet towels (or ice wrapped in a wet cloth) on the neck and forehead.

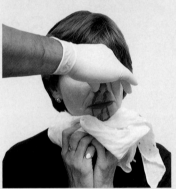

6   If bleeding persists, seek medical aid.

Other Wounds and Bleeding

BLEEDING FROM THE PALM

Bleeding from the palm may be severe as several blood vessels can be involved. There may also be damage to bones and nerves.

Management of Bleeding from Palm of Hand

1 Apply firm, direct pressure to palm —use a pad or something similar.

2 Bandage hand and fingers firmly —use a triangular or broad roller bandage.

3 Elevate hand in St John sling.

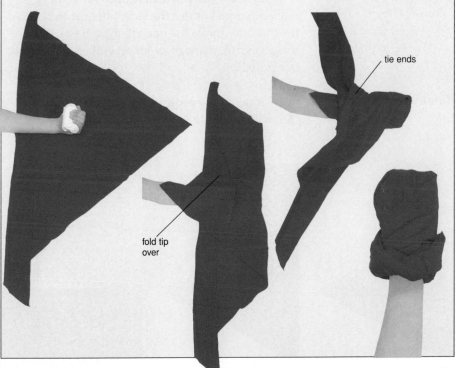

tie ends

fold tip over

To contain the bleeding and to apply pressure to the palm, you can use:

▶ a triangular bandage

▶ an unopened roller bandage

▶ a clean cloth wrapped around an object such as a matchbox or a smooth stone

▶ two or three fingers of the undamaged hand

A St John sling will elevate the hand to control the bleeding.

FISH HOOK WOUNDS

▶ do not remove fish hooks, except as detailed below

▶ seek medical aid

If aid is not readily available and the hook is embedded just under the skin, attempt to remove it—but only make the one attempt. If you are unsuccessful, manage as for an embedded object *(see p. 102)*.

Removal of fish hooks

1 If the barb is protruding, cut it off and withdraw the hook.

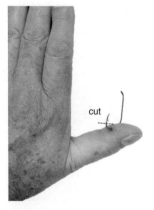
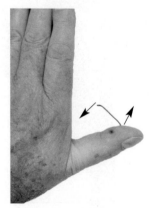
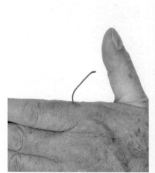

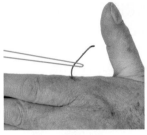

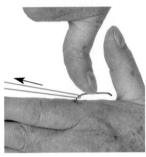

2 If the barb is embedded, loop fishing line along curve or throat of the hook and grip firmly in one hand.

3 Press down on the shank of the hook with thumb of other hand.

4 Pull the hook straight out.

5 Seek medical aid.

SPLINTER REMOVAL

Superficial splinters where the splinter end protrudes from the skin or is visible under the surface of the skin may be removed using the following procedure:

MANAGEMENT OF SPLINTER REMOVAL

1 Put on protective gloves—to minimize infection.

2 Clean the area around the splinter with soap and water.

3 If the splinter end protrudes from the skin–grasp the splinter with cleaned tweezers and remove the splinter at the angle it went in.

4 If the splinter end is **not** protruding from the skin— expose the splinter using a disposable sterile splinter probe and then remove as in Step 3.

5 Clean the area and apply a transparent or adhesive dressing.

6 Seek medical advice if:
• splinter area becomes more painful, reddened and swollen, or
• splinter breaks or does not come out easily.

BLEEDING FROM VARICOSE VEINS

The veins in the legs contain valves to keep the blood flowing towards the heart. When the valves deteriorate, blood leaks backwards and the pressure from the blood causes the vein to become swollen and knotted ('varicose'). They may bleed profusely if injured.

MANAGEMENT OF BLEEDING VARICOSE VEINS

1 Apply a clean pad and bandage firmly.

2 Place casualty flat with legs raised.

3 Remove any constricting items from limb.

4 Seek medical aid.

VAGINAL BLEEDING

If a woman is bleeding from the vagina, it is most likely to be associated with a monthly menstrual period. Ask the casualty if the bleeding is associated with her periods. Ask if she is pregnant. Vaginal bleeding in pregnancy must always be assumed to be serious.

MANAGEMENT OF VAGINAL BLEEDING

1 Take the woman to a private place.

2 Give her a sanitary pad or clean towel.

3 Make her comfortable—head and shoulders raised and supported, knees propped up.

4 **If the woman is possibly pregnant: ☎ *call 000 for an ambulance.***

If sexual assault has occurred or is suspected: Follow steps 1 to 3. Seek medical and police aid urgently. Stay with the casualty. Do not disturb evidence by removing, washing or disposing of clothing. If possible, persuade casualty not to go to toilet until a forensic examination has been carried out by a doctor.

INFECTION AND WOUNDS

Open wounds become infected as a result of micro-organisms entering the wound from the skin, the air or from germs on the object which caused the wound. Wounds are also likely to become infected if any foreign matter, dead tissue or bacteria remain in the wound.

A wound that has not begun to heal within two days may be infected. Infections can spread through the body and become life-threatening.

Signs of infection are

- increased pain and soreness
- increased temperature (warmth) around wound area
- increased swelling and redness of the wound and surrounding area
- pus oozing from the wound
- fever (if the infection persists)
- swelling and tenderness of the lymph glands

MANAGEMENT OF INFECTED WOUNDS

1 Dress wound with sterile bandage.

2 Elevate, if a limb, and immobilise.

3 Seek medical attention.

TETANUS

Tetanus is a potentially fatal disease caused by infection with the tetanus bacterium. The bacteria enter through an open wound and bacterial toxins affect the body's nervous system.

Signs and symptoms

- stiffness of the jaw (often the first sign)
- difficulty swallowing

▶ a stiff neck
▶ irritability and headaches
▶ chills and fever
▶ generalised stiffness
▶ spasms—local or general

Tetanus immunisation is effective for 10 years. Whenever any casualty sustains a wound ask if tetanus injection is current. If not, casualty should seek medical advice.

WOUNDS AND THE FIRST AIDER

If you have an open wound, laceration or ulcer, germs from the casualty's body fluids may more easily enter into your own body. Always have your own wounds covered and use disposable gloves whenever possible.

INTERNAL BLEEDING

Internal bleeding occurs when blood escapes from arteries, veins or capillaries into tissues or cavities in the body. Although capillary bleeding (indicated by mild bruising) is not serious, deeper bleeding involving veins and arteries may result in severe blood loss.

Severe internal bleeding usually results from injuries caused by a violent blunt force (such as in a car accident or fall from a height). It can also occur when an object (e.g. a knife) penetrates the skin and damages internal structures. Some conditions (such as a stomach ulcer or pregnancy) can also result in internal bleeding.

Internal bleeding can be as serious as external bleeding. Although there is no external loss of blood, blood is lost from the circulatory system and vital organs which may result in shock. Internal bleeding can also cause problems if it causes pressure on vital parts of the body such as the brain.

Signs and symptoms

- pain
- tenderness
- rigidity of abdominal muscles
- other signs of blood loss

Evidence of internal bleeding from some organs may be seen by the first aider. For example:
- coughing up red, frothy blood
- vomiting material which is obviously blood or may look like coffee grounds (coloured black)
- passing faeces with a black, tarry appearance

▶ passing faeces which are red in colour
▶ passing urine which has a red or smoky appearance

Internal bleeding may be accompanied by any of the signs and symptoms of major bleeding. Cardiac arrest can occur if enough blood is lost.

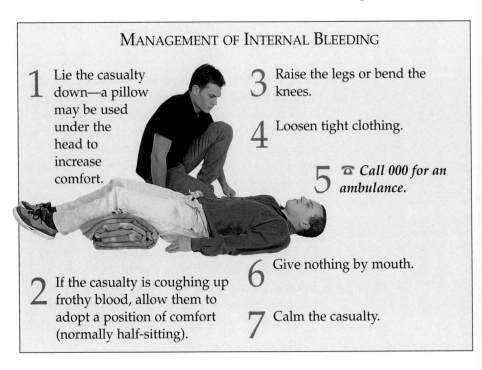

MANAGEMENT OF INTERNAL BLEEDING

1 Lie the casualty down—a pillow may be used under the head to increase comfort.

2 If the casualty is coughing up frothy blood, allow them to adopt a position of comfort (normally half-sitting).

3 Raise the legs or bend the knees.

4 Loosen tight clothing.

5 ☎ *Call 000 for an ambulance.*

6 Give nothing by mouth.

7 Calm the casualty.

PELVIC INJURIES

A pelvic injury is frequently the result of a car accident, a fall from a height or a crush injury. The casualty will feel pain in the region of the hips or groin which increases with movement. The casualty may be unable to stand and be aware of tenderness or bruising in the groin or scrotum. Signs of shock quickly develop.

MANAGEMENT OF PELVIC INJURIES

1 Follow DRABC.

2 Place casualty flat on back if conscious with knees bent and supported—a pillow may be used under the head to increase comfort.

3 Calm the casualty.

4 Remove contents of pockets (they can cause pressure and make movement painful).

5 ☎ *Call 000 for an ambulance.*

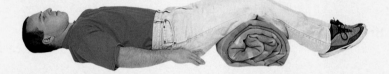

If medical aid will be delayed or you need to move the casualty:

1 Place soft padding between the knees, legs and ankles.

2 Apply a narrow figure of eight bandage around feet and ankles.

3 Apply a broad bandage around knees.

4 Support the pelvis on either side with rolled blankets or sandbags.

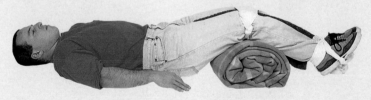

CRUSH INJURIES

A crush injury results when something large and heavy strikes or falls on a person. There are a number of situations in which this may occur: at a traffic accident, on a building site, at a train crash,

119

in an explosion, during an earthquake or in a mining accident.

Crush injuries are often very serious because of the damage they may cause: internal bleeding, fractured bones, ruptured organs and impaired circulation. If the casualty is trapped for any length of time, there is the risk of complications such as extensive tissue damage and shock, as well as the release of toxic substances into the circulation. This may lead, later, to acute kidney failure.

The first aider's aims

▶ ☎ *call 000 for an ambulance.*
▶ do whatever else is possible for the casualty

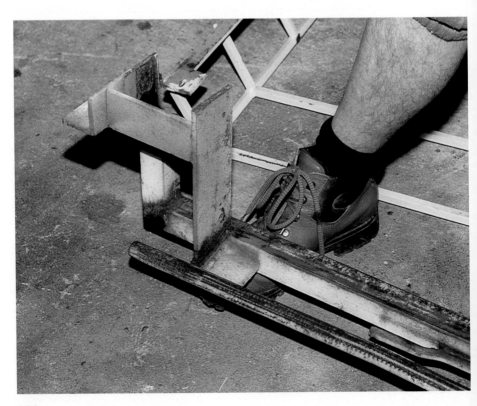

MANAGEMENT OF CRUSH INJURIES

1 Follow DRABC. DRABC

5 Control bleeding.

2 ☎ *Call 000 for an ambulance.*

6 Manage other injuries.

3 Ensure your own safety.

7 Comfort and reassure the casualty.

4 If safe remove the crushing object as quickly as possible.

HAEMATOMAS

A haematoma is caused by a sharp, blunt blow which does not break the skin but causes internal damage to blood vessels. This results in the accumulation of a quantity of blood at the site.

Signs and symptoms include

▶ severe pain
▶ area turning dark blue or red
▶ rapid and severe swelling
▶ loss of mobility of the area

A haematoma can be quite dangerous as it may conceal underlying injuries.

MANAGEMENT OF A HAEMATOMA

1 Follow DRABC.

DRABC

2 Follow RICE *(see p. 122).*

3 Seek medical aid.

RICE Management

R REST the casualty and the injured part.

I ICEPACKS (cold compress) wrapped in a cloth may be applied to the injury—for 15 minutes every 2 hours for 24 hours, then for 15 minutes every 4 hours for 24 hours.

C COMPRESSION BANDAGES, such as elastic bandages, should be firmly applied to extend well beyond the injury.

E ELEVATE the injured part.

Making a Cold Compress

A cold compress relieves pain and swelling by reducing the flow of blood to the injured area. It is usually left on the injury for 15 minutes at a time (as in RICE) and is changed whenever necessary to maintain the same level of coldness. It is usually left uncovered but can be secured with a gauze bandage or some other open-weave material.

Compresses can be made of:

▶ a cloth wrung out in cold water— needs replacing every 10 minutes

▶ a bag of frozen vegetables— wrapped in a light towel to protect the injury

▶ ice—in a sealed plastic bag two-thirds full of water, wrapped in a light towel

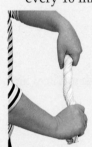
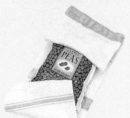
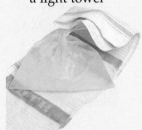

6

Fractures, dislocations, sprains and strains

Injuries to bones, joints and muscles are common. Although they are not usually life-threatening, they are painful. If not managed correctly they may cause lifelong disability and deformity.

In addition to the injury to bones, joints, ligaments and muscles, there may also be damage to the major blood vessels and nerves. As a result, there may be blood loss and shock, particularly if there are multiple injuries.

Appropriate first aid can reduce pain, shock and the risk of long-term complications from the injury.

This chapter includes the functions of bones, joints and muscles and the treatment of different types of bone, joint and muscle injuries.

THE MUSCULOSKELETAL SYSTEM

The musculoskeletal system is made up of various bones, muscles, tendons, ligaments and joints. It performs a number of functions such as providing support for the body, giving protection to internal organs, storing minerals, producing blood cells and enabling movement.

SKELETON

The skeleton is the internal framework of the body and is made up of 206 bones of various shapes and sizes. Its major functions are to support the skin and soft tissues of the body and to protect the vital organs (such as the heart, stomach and liver).

BONES

Bones are hard, dense, very strong structures and have an ample supply of blood and nerves. Some bones store and manufacture red blood cells in the bone marrow. Calcium is important for bone growth and repair. A lack of calcium in the diet can cause bones to weaken over time, because the body will use calcium from the bones for the body's other needs. A decrease in the calcium content of bones from about the age of 60 means bones can become frail, brittle and less dense and therefore more susceptible to fractures. This is called osteoporosis.

JOINTS

Joints are found wherever the bones meet. They are held together by ligaments. There are two types of joints: immovable and movable. Immovable joints are where the bones fit firmly

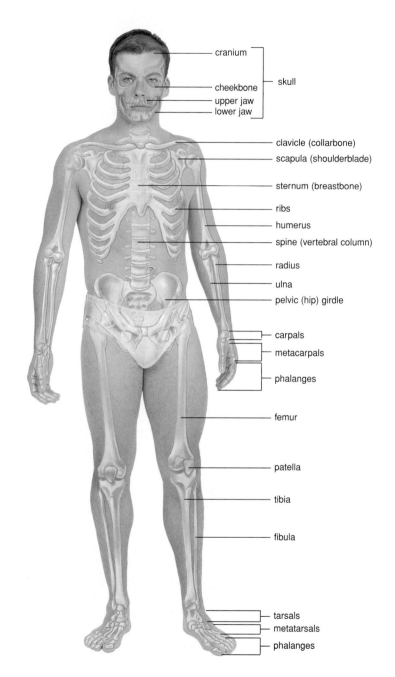

cranium

cheekbone

skull

upper jaw
lower jaw

clavicle (collarbone)

scapula (shoulderblade)

sternum (breastbone)

ribs

humerus

spine (vertebral column)

radius

ulna

pelvic (hip) girdle

carpals

metacarpals

phalanges

femur

patella

tibia

fibula

tarsals

metatarsals

phalanges

Human skeleton

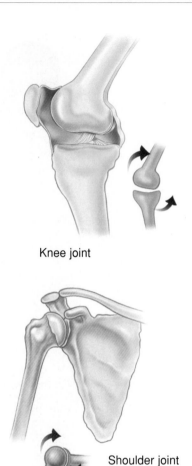

Knee joint

Shoulder joint

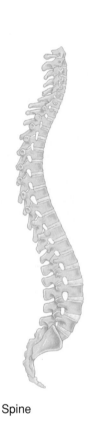

Spine

into each other or are fused (as in the skull). Some movable joints allow only slight movement (as between the vertebrae of the spine) while others allow a greater degree of movement (the ball-and-socket joint of the shoulder and the hinge joint in the knee). The amount of movement of the joint is restricted by the number of ligaments holding and supporting it. Joints with less support (fewer ligaments) are more prone to injury.

MUSCLES

Muscles are mostly, but not all, attached to bones by strong fibrous tissue called tendons. Muscles account for up to 50% of a person's body weight. By contracting and relaxing, the muscles pull the bones and this causes movement at the joints. Muscles are usually classed as voluntary or involuntary. Voluntary muscles are attached to the bones and are controlled by conscious messages from the brain. The involuntary muscles work continuously and automatically to operate internal organs such as the heart and stomach.

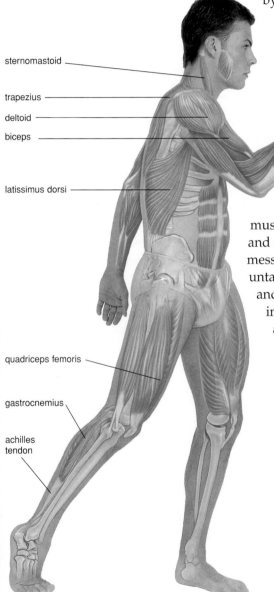

sternomastoid

trapezius

deltoid

biceps

latissimus dorsi

quadriceps femoris

gastrocnemius

achilles tendon

INJURIES TO THE MUSCULOSKELETAL SYSTEM

The bones in our body are built to withstand the many stresses placed on them. They are tough, dense and resilient but they can be broken (fractured) or displaced at a joint (dislocated).

Muscles, ligaments and tendons may be injured by being overstretched (as a result of a fall) or by being struck by something hard. This can result in a sprain (overstretching), a strain (torn muscle) or a bruise (internal bleeding from a blow) or a complete rupture.

Joints are injured when forced into a movement beyond their normal movement range.

Note: It can be difficult for a first aider to tell whether the injury is a fracture, dislocation, sprain or strain. If in doubt always treat as a fracture.

FRACTURES

A fracture is a break or crack in a bone. When a bone is broken there may be a single, clean break (simple fracture) or multiple bone fragments (complicated fracture). Bones may be chipped, cracked, or broken through.

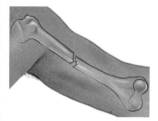

Simple fracture

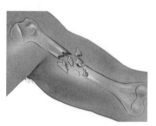

Complicated fracture

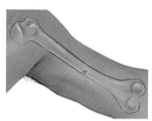

Greenstick fracture

In young children, bones are still growing and are more flexible and less likely to break than those of an adult. They may split, bend or crack just like a young tree branch and this is usually referred to as a 'greenstick fracture'.

Direct and indirect fractures

Fractures can be caused by either direct and indirect force. The bone can break at the point where it receives a heavy blow (direct fracture), or the force of the blow may travel from the point of impact through part of the body and cause a bone to fracture elsewhere (indirect fracture). For example, if a person falls and uses their hand to break the fall, the impact may travel along the arm and cause the collarbone to fracture.

Other indirect fractures can occur when a muscle pulls violently on an attached bone (such as when a golfer hits the ground instead of the golf ball) or

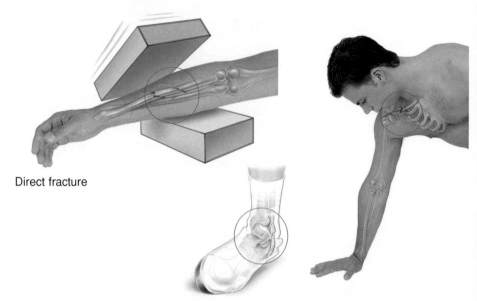

Direct fracture

Indirect fracture   Indirect fracture

when a twisting or wrenching force causes a
rotating strain to be transmitted to an attached
bone. This may occur if a person's ankle twists in
a fall and the strain causes the bones in that area
to fracture.

Complications   Any type of fracture can be complicated by injury
to adjoining muscles, blood vessels, nerves and
organs. Fractures of large bones can result in
considerable blood loss and shock.

Signs and symptoms
▶ pain at or near the site of injury
▶ tenderness at or near site of fracture
▶ swelling
▶ redness
▶ loss of function
▶ deformity
▶ casualty feels or hears the break occur
▶ a coarse grating sound is heard or felt as the
  bones rub against each other (crepitus)

TYPES OF FRACTURES

Fractures are classified as **closed, open** or **complicated.**

Closed

When a fracture is **closed**, the skin over the bone is not broken but there may be bleeding into surrounding tissues. Considerable damage may be done to surrounding muscles and blood vessels and there may be swelling in the affected area because of internal bleeding.

Open

In **open fractures**, the skin over the bone is broken and the bone may protrude through the skin. There is great danger of infection.

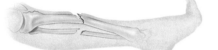 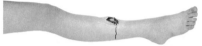

Complicated

Both open and closed fractures may be complicated when there is associated injury to a major nerve, blood vessels or vital organ (e.g. when a broken rib punctures a lung).

Remember: No attempt should be made to force a fracture back into place.

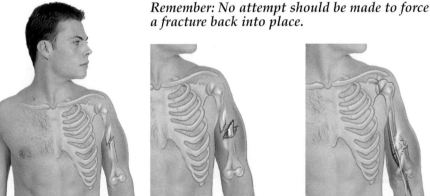
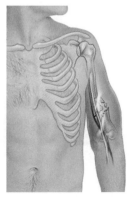

Closed fracture   Open fracture   Complicated fracture

131

A fracture involving a large bone or causing injury to a vital organ can cause marked distress either from heavy blood loss (internally or externally) or from damage to underlying organs.

Management

The main aim of management is to immobilise the injured part in order to lessen pain, reduce serious bleeding and shock, prevent further internal or external damage, and prevent a closed fracture becoming an open fracture.

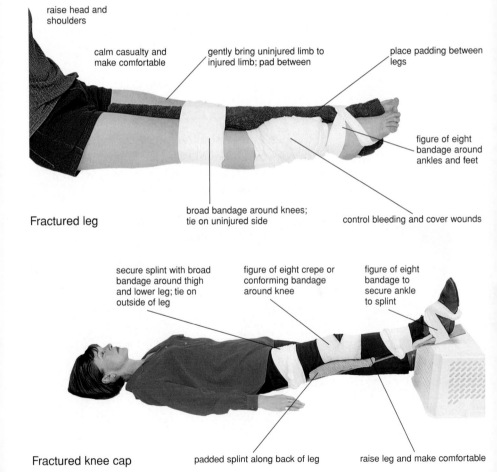

raise head and shoulders

calm casualty and make comfortable

gently bring uninjured limb to injured limb; pad between

place padding between legs

figure of eight bandage around ankles and feet

Fractured leg

broad bandage around knees; tie on uninjured side

control bleeding and cover wounds

secure splint with broad bandage around thigh and lower leg; tie on outside of leg

figure of eight crepe or conforming bandage around knee

figure of eight bandage to secure ankle to splint

Fractured knee cap

padded splint along back of leg

raise leg and make comfortable

MANAGEMENT OF A FRACTURE

1 Follow DRABC.

2 Control any bleeding and cover any wounds.

3 Check for fractures— open, closed or complicated.

4 Ask casualty not to move injured part.

5 Immobilise fracture with broad bandages (where possible) to prevent movement at the joints above and below the fracture:
- support the limb, carefully passing bandages under the natural hollows of the body
- place a padded splint along the injured limb (under leg for fractured kneecap)

- place padding between the splint and the natural contours of the body and secure tightly
- check that bandages not too tight (or too loose) every 15 minutes.

6 For leg fracture, immobilise feet and ankles with figure of eight bandage.

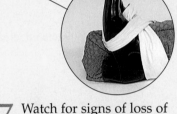

7 Watch for signs of loss of circulation to foot or hand (if possible).

8 Handle gently.

9 Observe casualty carefully.

10 Seek medical aid.

Note: If collarbone fractured, support arm on injured side in a St John sling.

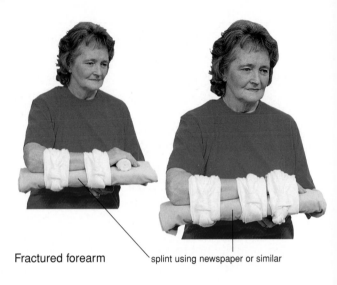

Fractured forearm — splint using newspaper or similar

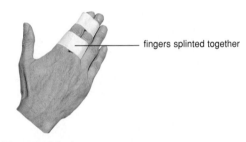

— fingers splinted together

Fractured finger

SPLINTS—GENERAL PRINCIPLES

1 Splint injury as close as possible to the anatomically correct position.

2 Make sure splint extends beyond the injured area (in both directions).

3 Apply broad bandages above and below fracture.

4 Immobilise joints above and below fracture.

5 Check circulation regularly— including in affected limb.

DISLOCATIONS

A dislocation occurs when one or more bones are displaced at a joint—at the shoulder, elbow, knee, wrist, ankle, hip or at the joints in the fingers and toes. This often occurs when a strong force acts directly or indirectly on the joint and wrenches the bone into an abnormal position. A dislocation can also be caused by a violent muscle contraction.

A dislocation can result in the ligaments in that area being torn. At times, the force may be strong enough to cause a fracture and damage nearby nerves and blood vessels.

Some joints, such as the shoulder or fingers, are more prone to dislocation because their ligaments provide less support than those in other joints, which dislocate less easily. A joint which is dislocated appears to be deformed because the dislocation causes an abnormal lump or depression. There may also be associated swelling.

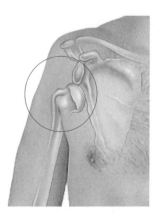 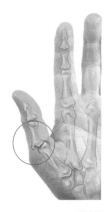

Signs and symptoms

▶ pain at or near the site of injury

▶ difficult or impossible normal movement

▶ loss of power

▶ deformity or abnormal mobility

▶ tenderness

▶ swelling

▶ discolouration and bruising

MANAGEMENT OF A DISLOCATION

Note: If in doubt, manage as a fracture.

1 Follow DRABC.

2 Do not attempt to reduce the dislocation.

3 **If a limb:**
- check circulation—
  if circulation absent move limb gently to try to restore it—otherwise do not move limb; ☎ *call 000 for an ambulance.*

- rest and support the limb using soft padding and bandages
- apply icepacks—if possible, directly to skin over joint

If a shoulder:
- support shoulder and arm in position of least discomfort and apply ice-packs.

SPRAINS

A sprain occurs when the ligaments and tissues holding together a joint are stretched and torn. This occurs when a joint is forced to move beyond its normal range. The more ligaments torn, the more severe the injury. Mild sprains, where the fibres of the ligaments are only stretched, will usually not take long to heal.

Pain from a sprain may be quite intense and the casualty's ability to move the joint will be restricted. There will be swelling around the joint and bruising will develop quickly.

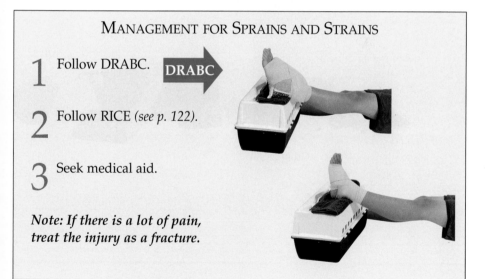

MANAGEMENT FOR SPRAINS AND STRAINS

1 Follow DRABC. **DRABC**

2 Follow RICE *(see p. 122).*

3 Seek medical aid.

Note: If there is a lot of pain, treat the injury as a fracture.

STRAINS

A strain occurs when the fibres of a muscle or tendon are stretched and torn. This usually happens as a result of lifting something too heavy, working a muscle too hard or making a sudden, uncoordinated movement. Common examples are the groin and hamstring strains of footballers. The casualty will feel sharp, sudden pain in the region of the injury and on any attempt to stretch the muscle. There is usually a loss of power in the affected limb and the muscle is tender.

Remember: If in doubt as to nature of injury, always treat as a fracture.

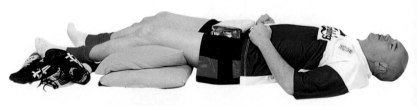

Groin strain

AMBULANCE ASSISTANCE

Ambulance or medical assistance must be sought for all fractures, and for other injuries when the person cannot move without assistance or is in significant pain.

An ambulance should be urgently called for a casualty when there is reduced circulation (limb pale and cold) or loss of sensation as a result of the injury.

Casualties who need an ambulance are:
- those in severe pain
- those who cannot use the affected limb
- those with a marked deformity of the limb or joint

Focus on Safety

Preventing Fractures and Dislocations

At home
- don't leave children unattended on or near stairs
- fit handrails on flights of steps and in showers and toilets
- use non-slip mats in wet areas

At work
- keep work areas tidy
- mark slippery areas clearly to warn others
- make sure carpet is laid properly and is not loose
- don't have rugs on slippery surfaces (e.g. tiles)
- make sure stairs are well lit and have handrails
- make sure ladders are stable before use

- wear safety belts and lifelines if working in high places

At sport
- avoid situations which may result in a fall
- do not travel at a speed which does not allow you to avoid sudden hazards
- learn how to cushion your body if you fall
- make sure there are no hazards in the sporting area which could cause a fall

On the road
- drive defensively
- use a seatbelt
- do not skylark

Preventing Sprains and Strains

- ensure your back is straight and knees bent when lifting
- if you are not sure you can lift a load or move a heavy object, don't try, get help

- warm up before exercising and don't push yourself beyond your limit

Chest and abdominal injuries

The chest and abdomen contain many of the body's major organs. The heart, lungs and major blood vessels around them are within the chest. Stomach, liver, pancreas, spleen, kidneys and intestines are in the abdomen.

Because of the importance of these organs, chest and abdominal injuries can be very serious and result in severe internal as well as external damage. The lungs are particularly vulnerable. Injury to the chest may result in a life-threatening situation with one or both lungs collapsing.

The chest and its organs are protected by the rib cage (12 pairs of ribs). The heart is protected by the breastbone (sternum) in front and by the vertebrae at the back. The chest is separated from the abdomen by a domed sheet of muscle (diaphragm). The rib cage gives some protection to the organs in the upper abdomen (liver and kidneys) but most abdominal organs are relatively unprotected by bones.

The chest and abdomen are therefore quite vulnerable, so injuries to these areas have to be treated carefully.

CHEST INJURIES

Chest injuries range from simple bruising, causing slight pain or discomfort during breathing, to life-threatening injury to the vital organs, seriously affecting breathing and circulation.

A wound or severe blow to the chest can interfere with breathing. If the wound penetrates the rib cage, air is able to enter the space occupied by the lungs. This results in one or both of the lungs collapsing. A wound to the lower chest can penetrate the abdominal area and cause severe internal injury.

Multiple fractures of the chest wall can cause a loss of rigidity, so that the rib cage does not move normally during breathing. This is called a flail chest.

A common cause of this type of injury is a road accident in which the driver is thrown against the steering wheel, or the steering column is pushed back into the driver's chest. The same type of injury can result if the chest is crushed by a heavy object.

OPEN AND CLOSED INJURIES

Open

Chest injuries can be open or closed. In an open chest injury the skin has been punctured as a result of either an external object or a broken rib penetrating the chest wall.

Closed

In a closed chest injury, the skin of the chest has not been broken. Although there may not be any visible sign of injury, there could be serious damage (bruising or rupture) to internal organs and tissues.

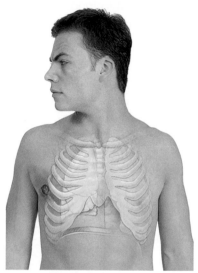

Open chest injury

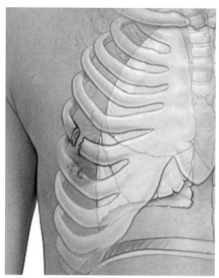

Closed chest injury

Types of injury	Examples of causes
• fractured ribs	• blows (e.g. steering wheel impact)
• flail chest *(see p. 147)*	• falls
• bruising of the lung	• crushing by heavy objects
• penetrating chest wound	• stabbing
• lung injury (e.g. bleeding, collapse of the lung, leaking of air and/or blood into the chest space)	• gunshots
	• blasts

Assessing a chest injury

Make a careful examination of the chest area if the casualty is having trouble breathing or complains of pain in the chest area, and the possible cause suggests a chest injury.

▶ expose the chest area (try to ensure privacy for a female casualty)

▶ look for signs of broken ribs, local tenderness or a wound

▶ look for bruises, deformity, blood and abnormal chest movement while breathing

COLLAPSED LUNG (PNEUMOTHORAX)

Traumatic pneumothorax

Wounds which penetrate the chest can range from minor to life-threatening. If a puncture is deep enough the rib cage may be penetrated, allowing air to enter the chest through the wound. When air enters this space (pleural cavity), the lung on the side of the injury collapses. This is called an open or traumatic pneumothorax.

MANAGEMENT OF A TRAUMATIC PNEUMOTHORAX

Manage as for a penetrating chest wound *(see p. 149)*.

Spontaneous pneumothorax

A closed or spontaneous pneumothorax may happen in otherwise healthy people without any apparent cause. It can be the result of a violent bout of coughing, a severe asthma attack, a serious lung infection or a broken rib piercing the lung.

Signs and symptoms

▶ pain (often under the shoulderblade) on the affected side, whenever the casualty breathes

▶ difficulty breathing

▶ restricted or no movement of chest wall on the affected side

▶ rapid, weak pulse

A pneumothorax can involve the collapse of one or both lungs, resulting in a life-threatening situation. The first aider cannot stop the build-up of air in the pleural cavity.

MANAGEMENT OF A SPONTANEOUS PNEUMOTHORAX

1 Follow DRABC.

2 ☎ *Call 000 for an ambulance.*

3 Make the casualty as comfortable as possible.

4 Calm the casualty.

5 Complete the initial assessment.

6 Monitor vital signs.

7 Give emergency care as required.

FRACTURED RIBS

A simple rib fracture is rarely life-threatening but is painful. In a more serious fracture, the ribs may be forced into the lungs, causing damage. As a result, blood and air may collect in the chest space.

The casualty will usually attempt to ease the pain by supporting the injured area with the hand or arm. Breathing will be difficult and usually shallow, because normal or deep breathing is painful.

Signs and symptoms

▶ pain (worsens when the casualty breathes or coughs)
▶ tenderness at site of injury
▶ short, rapid breathing
▶ frothy, bloodstained sputum

Management of Fractured Ribs

Conscious casualty

1   Place in a comfortable position (normally half-sitting and leaning to the injured side, if other injuries permit).

2   Encourage the casualty to breathe with short breaths.

3   Gently place ample padding over the injured area.

4   Apply one or two broad bandages (depending on size of casualty), securing arm and padding to chest on injured side.

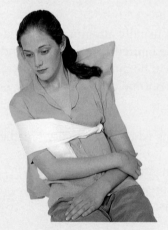

5   Tie bandages in front on uninjured side.

6   If bandages increase discomfort, loosen or remove them.

7   Immobilise the arm using a St John sling or collar and cuff sling.

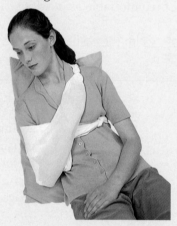

8   ☎ *Call 000 for an ambulance.*

Unconscious casualty

1   Follow DRABC.

2   Lie casualty on injured side, in recovery position.

3   ☎ *Call 000 for an ambulance.*

PENETRATING CHEST WOUND

A penetrating chest wound can cause severe internal damage within both the chest and upper abdomen. The lungs are particularly vulnerable to injury. Even if they are not punctured, air could enter the chest cavity. This exerts pressure on the lung and may cause it to collapse. Pressure in the chest cavity may build up to such an extent that the heart is pushed to the side. Thus the function of the uninjured lung on that side may also be affected. The build-up of pressure may also prevent adequate refilling of the heart, impairing the circulation and causing shock.

The aims of management

▶   seal wound, allow fluid and air to escape from wound and maintain breathing
▶   ☎ *call 000 for an ambulance.*

Signs and symptoms

▶   pain at site of wound
▶   unconsciousnes
▶   difficult and painful breathing
▶   bloodstained bubbles around wound when casualty exhales
▶   sound of air being sucked into chest as the casualty inhales

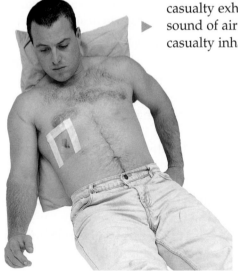

How to cover a penetrating chest wound

MANAGEMENT OF A PENETRATING CHEST WOUND

1 Follow DRABC.

DRABC►

2 Place casualty in whatever position makes breathing easiest.

3 Cover the wound—use the casualty's or your own hand (to stop air flowing in and out of chest cavity).

4 Cover wound with a dressing (such as plastic sheet, bag or aluminium foil)—if not available, use a sterile dressing or pad.

5 Seal with tape on three sides (not bottom).

6 ☎ *Call 000 for an ambulance.*

FLAIL CHEST

A flail chest occurs when a number of ribs in the same area are broken so that part of the chest is 'floating free'. The injured part of the chest wall is called the 'flail' or 'loose' segment. It does not move with the rest of the rib cage when the casualty breathes. Instead it moves in the opposite direction. This is called **paradoxical breathing**.

If many of the ribs are broken (as can happen when the chest hits the steering wheel in a car accident), the whole breastbone can become a flail segment. Breathing becomes difficult because of the pain and tissue damage.

Signs and symptoms

▶ difficulty in breathing and shortness of breath (gasping for air)
▶ chest pain
▶ blue colouring of the mouth, nailbeds and skin
▶ difficulty in speaking
▶ the loose part moving in a direction opposite to that of normal breathing
▶ possible unconsciousness

MANAGEMENT OF A FLAIL CHEST

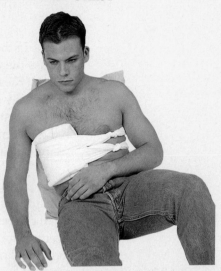

1 Follow DRABC.

DRABC

2 **If casualty conscious**, place casualty in a comfortable position (normally half-sitting, leaning to the injured side).

If casualty unconscious, turn to the injured side, in recovery position.

3 Loosen tight clothing.

4 Place a large bulky dressing over the loose area with a firm bandage.

5 Bend arm on injured side at elbow and, with fingers pointing to opposite shoulder, securely bandage to chest.

6 ☎ *Call 000 for an ambulance.*

ABDOMINAL INJURIES

Organs in the abdomen can easily be injured because there is no bone structure to protect them. Some of these—liver, spleen and stomach—tend to bleed easily and profusely, so injuries to them can be life-threatening. Injury to the bowel may result in the contents being spilled into the abdominal cavity, causing infection.

An injury to the abdomen can be open or closed. Both are serious as even in a closed wound an organ can be ruptured, causing serious internal bleeding and shock. With an open injury, abdominal organs can protrude through the wound.

Signs and symptoms

▶ severe pain
▶ nausea or vomiting
▶ bruising and tenderness around the wound
▶ unnatural paleness
▶ external bleeding
▶ blood in the urine
    ▶ protrusion of intestines through an abdominal wound
       ▶ shock

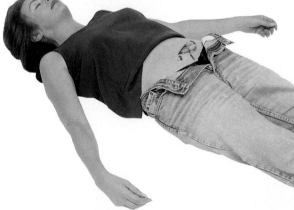

MANAGEMENT OF ABDOMINAL INJURIES

1 Follow DRABC.

DRABC

2 Place casualty on back with knees slightly raised and supported—a pillow may be used under the head to increase comfort.

3 Loosen clothing.

4 Cover protruding organs with aluminium foil or plastic food wrap, or a large, non-stick, sterile dressing, soaked in sterile saline (clean water if saline not available).

5 Secure with broad bandage (not tightly).

6 ☎ *Call 000 for an ambulance.*

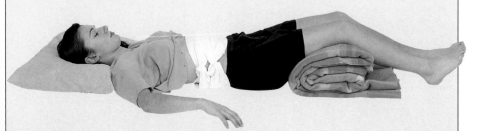

DO NOT give anything to drink.
DO NOT try to push organs back into abdomen.
DO NOT apply direct pressure to the wound.

Chapter

Head, neck and spinal injuries

8

The seriousness of injuries to the head, neck and spine cannot be overstated. Once the brain or spinal cord is damaged, the damage may be permanent. The brain and spinal cord do not regenerate themselves after injury—nerve cells are not renewed.

Damage to the brain or spinal cord is one of the most disabling traumatic conditions. Injuries to the head can be complicated by unconsciousness—a sign there is significant brain injury and risk of further injury. Injury to the spine will interfere with the transmission of messages to and from the brain, so that parts of the body may be paralysed and without sensation.

Any casualty with a head or spinal injury, including injury to the neck, must receive medical aid urgently. This chapter outlines what help the first aider can give.

HEAD AND SPINAL COLUMN

Skull

The skull gives the head its shape and protects the brain. It is made up of:
- plate-like bones which fuse together during childhood to form a rigid structure (cranium)
- facial bones which join with the cranium to form the eye and nose cavities
- upper and lower jaws

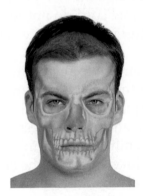 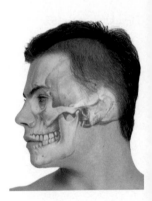

Spine

The spine is a flexible column consisting of 33 small bones called vertebrae aligned one on top of the other. Between the vertebrae are flexible discs which act as shock absorbers for the spine. Each vertebra has an opening in the centre forming a channel from the top to the bottom of the spine.

Spinal cord

The spinal cord runs through the channel and is protected by the spine. It is entirely encased within the spine, floating in a bag of fluid, called cerebrospinal fluid. This cushions the stresses of movement. The spinal cord is a continuation of the brain, its nerves radiating out into the rest of the body. The spinal cord and nerves carry

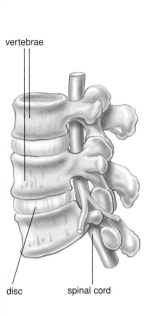

vertebrae

disc   spinal cord

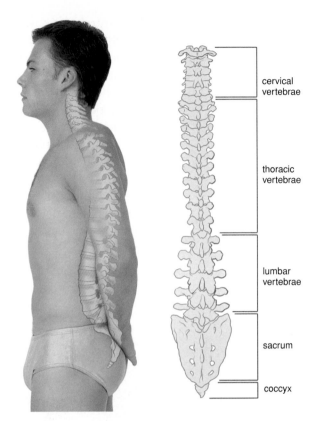

cervical
vertebrae

thoracic
vertebrae

lumbar
vertebrae

sacrum

coccyx

messages, as electrical impulses, from the brain to the rest of the body and from the body back to the brain. The spine may be injured anywhere along its length, threatening the spinal cord.

If the spine is injured, the vertebrae may be fractured and the ligaments sprained. These injuries usually heal without complications. However, severe injuries to the spinal cord itself can result in complete and permanent loss of feeling, and paralysis below the point where the injury occurred. The casualty may become a paraplegic (paralysed from the waist down) or a quadriplegic (paralysed from the neck down).

Nervous system

The central nervous system consists of the brain and the spinal cord, both of which are protected by the cerebrospinal fluid. The central nervous system contrasts with the peripheral nervous system which is made up of:

▶ 12 pairs of cranial nerves arising directly from the brain

▶ 31 pairs of spinal nerves running from the spinal cord throughout the body

The autonomic nervous system, which is part of the peripheral nervous system, controls automatic functions such as heartbeat, digestion and sweating.

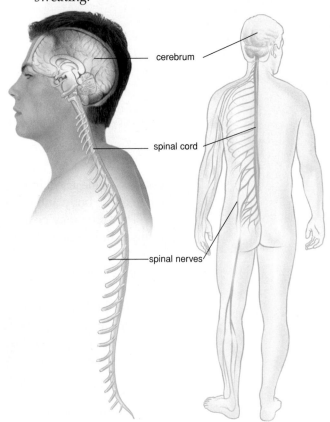

cerebrum

spinal cord

spinal nerves

HEAD INJURIES

Because the brain is the controlling organ for the whole body, injuries to the head are potentially dangerous and always require medical attention. When a casualty has a serious head injury, the neck or spine may also be injured.

> **Warning**
>
> If casualty is—or becomes—unconscious, suspect a spinal injury. Take extreme care to maintain spine alignment; immobilise as soon as possible.

Fractures

Fractures may occur in the cranium, at the base of the skull, or in the face. The skull may be fractured by a direct force (e.g. a blow to the head) or indirect force (e.g. a fall from a height, landing heavily on the feet). Severe injuries may cause multiple cracking (an 'eggshell' fracture) which may extend to the base of the skull.

Concussion

Concussion is an altered state of consciousness, usually caused by a blow to the head or neck. The casualty may become unconscious but this is often momentary. Common causes are car accidents, falls and sports injuries. The casualty usually recovers quickly but there is always the possibility of serious brain injury.

Compression

Compression is excess pressure on part of the brain. It may be caused by a depressed skull fracture where the broken bones put pressure on the brain, or by a build-up of fluids in the skull. If a blow to the head causes bleeding in the brain and the blood cannot drain from the closed space, it builds up and puts pressure on the brain. This is life-threatening.

157

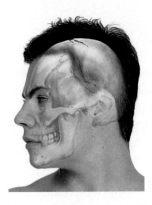

ASSESSMENT OF HEAD INJURIES

It is often very difficult to make an accurate assessment of the severity of a head injury. Therefore no head injury should be disregarded or treated lightly. As there is the possibility that complications will develop later, the casualty should always be advised to seek medical aid.

The cause of the injury is often the best indication of its severity. Strong forces will usually cause severe injuries to the head and spine (e.g. being thrown through the window of a car in a high-speed accident).

Signs and symptoms

Depending on where the injury is, blood may appear from the ears or nose. If the base of the skull is fractured there may be no obvious sign of injury, but cerebrospinal fluid or blood may escape through the ears.

If the casualty temporarily loses consciousness yet does not have any apparent injury or after-effects, the first aider should assume the potential for hidden injury. Advise the casualty to seek medical aid promptly. Signs and symptoms of head injury include:

- headache
- loss of memory (amnesia), particularly of the event
- altered or abnormal responses to commands and touch
- wounds to the scalp or to face

In more complicated cases, signs and symptoms include:

- blood or clear fluid escaping from nose or ears
- pupils becoming unequal in size
- blurred vision

MANAGEMENT OF HEAD INJURIES

1 Follow DRABC.

2 Manage casualty as if unconscious:
- place in recovery position
- clear and open airway
- monitor breathing and circulation.

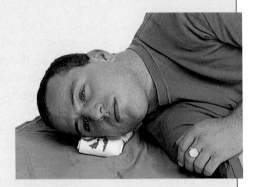

3 Support casualty's head and neck during movement; avoid twisting movement (could have spinal injury).

4 Keep casualty's airway open with your fingers if face badly injured (do not force).

5 Control bleeding but do not apply direct pressure to the skull if you suspect a fracture.

6 If blood or fluid comes from the ear, cover with a sterile dressing (lie casualty on injured side if possible to allow fluid to drain).

7 Lightly cover an eye injury with a sterile pad.

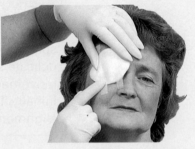

8 ☎ *Call 000 for an ambulance.*

Warning

An unconscious casualty with a head injury may vomit. Be ready to turn casualty onto the side, supporting head and neck, and clear the airway quickly. You will need at least one helper to do this successfully.

Spinal Injuries

A spinal cord injury is particularly traumatic because the resulting damage may be permanent. Adolescents and young adults tend to be the main casualties.

Spinal injuries are always serious and must be treated with great care. Incorrect handling of a casualty can result in paralysis. Careful assessment and management will help minimise permanent disability and increase the casualty's potential for recovery.

> **Warning**
>
> Twisting, compressing or bending an injured spine may worsen damage. Damage to the delicate spinal cord may occur as a result of movement, even if the cord was not injured initially. Take extreme care to maintain alignment of spine.

If the spinal cord is damaged, no messages will be received by the brain, or sent to that part of the body below the injury. The control centres for breathing and heart are in the lower parts of the brain and in the upper spinal cord. Death may result if these vital cell groups are damaged or if their messages cannot pass an injured section of the spinal cord.

Remember: After DRABC, swift immobilisation is the highest priority for all spinal injuries.

Causes of spinal injuries

▶ falls from a height
▶ direct blow to the spine
▶ penetrating injury such as gunshot or knife wound
▶ diving or surfing accidents
▶ high-speed accidents
▶ sudden acceleration or deceleration injuries (such as whiplash)
▶ being thrown from a vehicle or motorcycle
▶ pedestrian being hit by vehicle
▶ being hit from above by falling objects

Signs and symptoms

▶ pain at or below site of injury
▶ tenderness over site of injury
▶ absent or altered sensation (e.g. tingling in hands or feet)
▶ loss of movement or impaired movement below site of injury

If the casualty is unconscious as a result of a head injury, the first aider should always suspect a spinal injury.

MANAGEMENT OF SPINAL INJURIES

Immobilising the spine is the priority for any casualty with a suspected spinal injury. If the casualty is conscious and medical aid is only minutes away—as in urban areas—place something fairly solid (e.g. an article of clothing, sandbag, padded rock) on either side of the casualty's head to prevent movement of the neck and spine.

If the casualty is unconscious, the airway must be kept open. Remember, airway, breathing and circulation (ABC) always take precedence. The casualty should be placed in the recovery position, extreme care being taken to maintain alignment of the spine so as to avoid aggravating any possible neck or spinal injury.

NECK INJURIES

Management of neck injuries

As the upper spine is part of the neck, all management points for spinal injuries are also relevant for neck injuries. Manage as for spinal injury.

MANAGEMENT OF SPINAL INJURIES (INCLUDING NECK)

Unconscious casualty with suspected spinal injury

1   Follow DRABC. **DRABC**

2   Place casualty in recovery position supporting neck and spine at all times.

3   Maintain a clear and open airway.

4   Hold head and spine steady with supports, to prevent twisting or bending movement.

5   Apply a cervical or improvised collar (if possible) to minimise neck movement.

6   ☎ *Call 000 for an ambulance.*

Conscious casualty with suspected spinal injury

1   Calm the casualty.

2   Loosen tight clothing.

3   **DO NOT MOVE** casualty unless in danger—leave lifting, loading and transporting casualty to qualified personnel (e.g. ambulance officer) unless absolutely necessary.

4   Support head and neck—place your hands on either side of casualty's head until other support arranged.

5 Hold head and spine steady with supports.

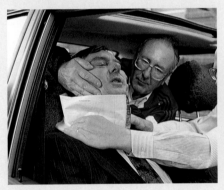

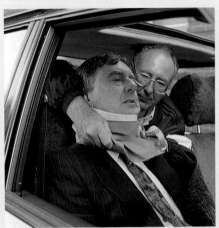

6 Apply a cervical collar if available (a folded towel, newspaper or other bulky dressing can be used if collar not available).

7 ☎ *Call 000 for an ambulance.*

Remember: Take extreme care at all times to maintain alignment of neck and spine.

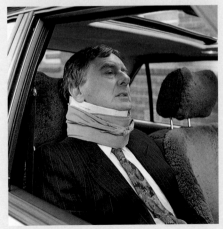

Focus on Safety

Preventing Head, Neck and Spinal Injuries

At home
- make sure floors are not slippery—mop up spilt liquids and clean up grease on floors immediately
- don't have rugs on slippery surfaces (e.g. tiles)
- use ladders with care

At work
- wear safety belts and lifelines if working in high places
- wear a 'hard hat' in specified workplaces
- make sure any structure on which you are working is firmly secured
- use a tractor with caution, especially on slopes or pulling a load

At sport
- inspect playground equipment periodically
- remain well clear of someone swinging a bat, golf club or racquet
- don't dive into shallow water or where depth is unknown
- wear a helmet for cricket, and horse riding

On the road
- drive defensively and avoid unsafe driving practices
- use seatbelts (children in correct restraint for age)
- wear a helmet if riding a motorcycle or bicycle

Eye injuries

9

So much of what we do and how we operate in our environment assumes the ability to see—loss of sight can therefore be a devastating experience. The eye can be injured very easily.

Eye injuries can be caused in many ways— by blunt blows; by trauma from fingernails or cuts by paper; by foreign objects such as soot or grit entering the eye; by damage from burning fluids or chemicals; and by the effects of light or radiant energy. Eyes are injured in the home, at work, at sport and in road accidents.

The first aider has a very important role in ensuring that first aid is given immediately to minimise the chances of partial or complete loss of sight. In a number of cases, it will be necessary to seek medical aid as quickly as possible.

EYE INJURIES

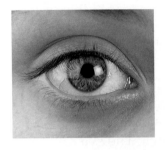

The eye is one of the most sensitive and delicate organs in the body. It is easily injured so it is important to treat the eye with great care. Infection can result in later damage to eyesight. Any eye injury can be serious because it can damage the cornea, the transparent tissue forming the circular lens in front of the eye. One rule of first aid for eye injuries is to prevent scratching of, or further damage to, the cornea.

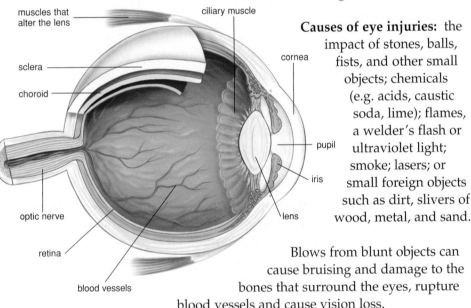

muscles that alter the lens
ciliary muscle
sclera
cornea
choroid
pupil
iris
optic nerve
lens
retina
blood vessels

Causes of eye injuries: the impact of stones, balls, fists, and other small objects; chemicals (e.g. acids, caustic soda, lime); flames, a welder's flash or ultraviolet light; smoke; lasers; or small foreign objects such as dirt, slivers of wood, metal, and sand.

Blows from blunt objects can cause bruising and damage to the bones that surround the eyes, rupture blood vessels and cause vision loss.

Foreign objects can be irritating, and cause a great deal of pain and significant damage. The eye tries to flush the foreign object out by producing tears, but this is not always successful. It may be necessary to take further action to remove the object.

Any sharp object which penetrates the eyeball can cause serious damage and will cause infection if not properly managed.

EXAMINATION OF EYE INJURIES

Inspection of the eye may be difficult because of spasm, swelling, or twitching; mucus and blood discharge; or injuries to eyelid or face.

An eye injury always results in pain and 'watering'. The 'whites of the eye' become red. The casualty may be unable to open the eye.

If the casualty wears contact lenses and they can be removed easily, ask the casualty to remove them before you deal with the eye injury. Do not remove the lenses yourself. A contact lens should not be removed if the surface of the eye is badly injured.

General principles for managing eye injuries

1 Wash hands thoroughly and put gloves on—remove any powder from gloves by washing.

2 **DO NOT** attempt to remove an object which is embedded in the eye or is on the coloured part of the eye.

3 Cover injured eye with sterile pad.

4 Never put direct pressure on eyeball.

5 Seek medical aid quickly.

TYPES OF EYE INJURIES

FOREIGN OBJECTS IN THE EYE

Loose eyelashes, grit, dust, glass, cosmetics, metal particles, and insects are some of the foreign objects that may enter the eye.

Warn the casualty of the importance of NOT rubbing the eye, even if the desire to do so is very strong. Rubbing may damage the cornea or other parts of the eye.

DO NOT remove a foreign object from the cornea.
DO NOT remove any object embedded in the eye.
DO NOT persist in examining the eye if the injury is severe.

Management of a Foreign Object in the Eye

If the object is small and is not embedded in the eye, it may be washed out by natural 'watering' (tears). If tears do not rid the eye of the foreign object:

1 Ask casualty to look up.

2 Gently draw the lower lid down and out.

3 **If object visible:**
   • remove using corner of a clean, moist cloth

   If object not visible:
   • ask casualty to look down
   • gently grasp lashes of upper lid

   • pull lid down and over lower lid. This may dislodge the foreign object.

If unsuccessful:

4 Wash eye with gentle stream of sterile saline or clean water.

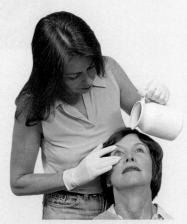

If all unsuccessful:

5 Lie casualty down.

6 Place thick pads above and below the injured eye.

7 Cover injured eye, making sure pads do not press on the eye.

8 Seek medical aid.

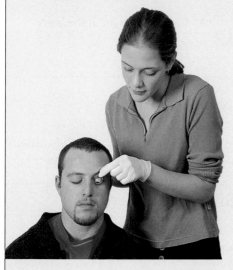

WOUNDS TO THE EYE

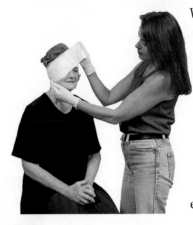

Wounds to the eye caused by a direct blow (e.g. in a fist fight) or by fast moving objects (e.g. a squash ball) can be painful and severe. If the injury is severe, do not persist in examining the eye.

MANAGEMENT OF WOUNDS TO THE EYE

1 Follow DRABC.

2 Calm casualty.

3 Place dressing over injured eye (make sure there is no pressure on eye).

4 Ask casualty not to move eyes.

5 Lie casualty on back.

6 ☎ *Call 000 for an ambulance.*

SMOKE IN THE EYES

Smoke in the eyes will probably cause the casualty pain and the eyes will look red and watery.

MANAGEMENT OF SMOKE IN THE EYES

1 Follow DRABC.

2 Ask casualty not to rub eyes.

3 Wash eyes with sterile saline or cold tap water.

BURNS TO THE EYE

Causes

▶ chemicals (e.g. acids, caustic soda, lime, plant juices or sap)
▶ heat (flames or radiant heat)
▶ welding flash or other ultraviolet light
▶ glues and solvents

In addition to the eyes being painful, red and very watery, they will be sensitive to light and eyelids will be swollen. If the injury has been caused by welder's flash, the eyes will feel gritty and painful. This is not felt until several hours after the exposure. The eyelids are often in spasm. Snow blindness is also caused by ultraviolet light, and symptoms are the same as those caused by welder's flash.

If chemicals have burnt the eye, immediate action must be taken.

MANAGEMENT OF BURNS TO THE EYE

Chemical or heat burn

1 Follow DRABC.

2 Open eyelids gently.

3 Wash eye gently with cold flowing water for at least 20 minutes (make sure to wash under eyelids).

4 Place eye pad or light clean dressing over injured eye.

5 ☎ *Call 000 for an ambulance.*

Welder's flash, snow blindness or other ultraviolet light burn

1 Place eye pads or light clean dressings over the injured eyes.

2 Seek medical aid.

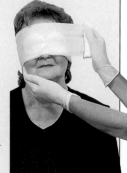

171

EMBEDDED OBJECT IN EYE

A first aider should never try to remove any object embedded in the eye.

Note: Vomiting makes penetrating eye injuries worse, due to the increased pressure caused by retching.

LACERATIONS AND BRUISES AROUND THE EYE

Lacerated eyelids generally bleed profusely because of the many blood vessels in this area. A dressing on the injured part will usually control bleeding. However care must be taken to make sure there is no pressure applied to the eyeball as this may cause permanent damage.

MANAGEMENT OF EYE INJURIES

Small foreign object in eye	Wounds to the eye
DRABC	DRABC
Ask casualty to look up. Draw lower eyelid down. If object visible, use corner of moistened clean cloth to remove it.	Place light dressing over injured eye.
If not visible, pull upper lid down to dislodge object.	Lie casualty in comfortable position on back.
If unsuccessful, wash eye with gentle stream of sterile saline or clean water.	Ask casualty not to move eyes.
If still unsuccessful, lie casualty in comfortable position on back.	Seek medical aid.
Seek medical aid.	

Management of an Embedded Object in the Eye

1 Follow DRABC.

2 Lie casualty on back.

3 **DO NOT** attempt to remove object.

4 Place pads around the object or paper cup over it.

5 Bandage in place.

6 ☎ *Call 000 for an ambulance.*

7 **DO NOT** give any food or drink

lie casualty in comfortable position

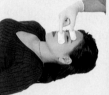
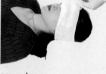
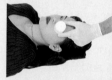
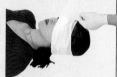

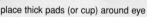

place thick pads (or cup) around eye

ensure there is no pressure on eye

Smoke in the eyes	**Burns to the eye**	**Embedded object in eye**
DRABC	DRABC	DRABC
		Lie casualty in comfort able position on back.
Ask casualty not to rub eyes.	Open eyelids gently and wash eye with cold flowing water for 20 mins.	Place thick pads above and below eye or cover object with paper cup.
Wash eyes with sterile saline or cold tap water.	Place eye pad or light clean dressing over injured eye.	Bandage pads in place making sure there is no pressure on eyelids.
Seek medical aid if necessary.	Seek medical aid.	Seek medical aid.

FOCUS ON SAFETY

PREVENTING EYE INJURIES

- never allow a child or other person to stand near a work-bench when in use if slivers of material may fly out (e.g. woodturning, metal working)
- wear eye protection when working in an environment where small objects may fly around
- wear protective eye wear on a building site or other dangerous work site
- pick up stones and other similar materials before commencing mowing
- stay clear of someone chopping wood
- wear protective eye wear when playing sports in which eye injuries are common (e.g. squash)
- make sure there is no-one between you and the target when playing sports such as darts, archery or shooting

10

Medical emergencies

Asthma, diabetes and epilepsy affect a significant proportion of Australia's population. The incidence of asthma in Australia and New Zealand is the highest in the world.

An asthma attack can be life-threatening. An epileptic seizure can be frightening for someone untrained to deal with it.

A significant proportion of the Australian population is known to be allergic to specific triggers. Allergy triggers include certain foods, insect bites and stings, and some prescribed or non-prescribed drugs. If an allergic reaction is very severe, the casualty may suffer anaphylactic shock, which is life-threatening.

Other medical emergencies include convulsions and fainting.

This chapter looks at the role of the first aider in each of these situations.

MEDICAL EMERGENCIES

People live with conditions such as asthma, diabetes and epilepsy without a noticeable effect on their lifestyles. However, a medical emergency can arise unexpectedly from complications of these disorders. The cause is not always immediately evident. In such an emergency, the first aider will respond using the DRABC Action Plan and appropriate care.

It is often difficult for the first aider to decide when to send for emergency medical help. If the problem does not resolve itself quickly or you have doubts about its severity, it is better to err on the side of caution and call 000 for an ambulance.

If you are faced with someone who suddenly suffers a diabetic emergency, has an epileptic or other seizure, faints, or has an asthma attack, some general guidelines should be followed.

GENERAL PRINCIPLES FOR MANAGEMENT OF MEDICAL EMERGENCIES

1 Follow DRABC. **DRABC**

2 Prevent further injury.

3 Monitor the airway, breathing and circulation.

4 When necessary:
☎ *call 000 for an ambulance.*

5 Provide reassurance.

6 Provide any specific care that will help the condition.

7 Help the casualty to rest comfortably.

Asthma

Asthma is a condition in which the bronchi (air tubes of the lungs) go into spasm and become narrower. Excess mucus is produced, causing the person to have difficulty breathing. Asthma is particularly common in children.

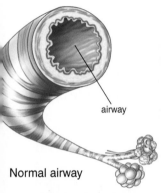

Normal airway

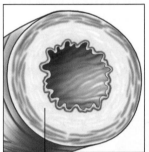

trigger factors lead to inflammation

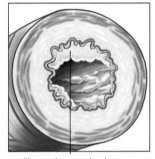

swelling and mucus in airway

Asthma affected airways

Signs and symptoms

The casualty may be:
- unable to get enough air
- progressively more anxious, short of breath, subdued or panicky
- focused only on breathing
- coughing, wheezing
- pale, sweating
- blue around lips, ear lobes and fingertips
- unconscious

Note: A wheeze may be audible. However, in a severe attack there may be so little air movement that a wheeze may not be heard.

When to send for medical aid

- if breathing does not become easier soon after medication—within 4 minutes
- the attack increases in severity

177

MEDICATION

Asthmatics use two types of medication—relievers and preventers.

Relievers

Relievers open the narrowed airways. They act within seconds or minutes. First aiders are primarily involved with relievers in the acute or emergency situation. If an asthma attack occurs, the reliever, usually in a blue or grey container, is taken to provide relief. Relievers reduce the spasm and open the bronchi to allow oxygen to be taken up.

Preventers

Preventers stop attacks or reduce severity if they 'break through'. Preventers are usually in a brown or yellow container. This form of medication must be taken regularly to prevent asthma attacks.

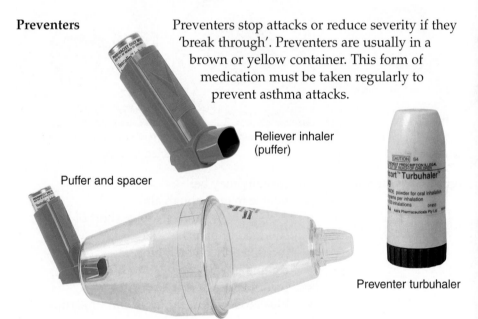

Reliever inhaler
(puffer)

Puffer and spacer

Preventer turbuhaler

Administration

These medications are given via a 'puffer', a small pressure canister which releases a regulated dose into the mouth when the canister is pressed. Sometimes a puffer is used in conjunction with a 'spacer' device. Medication may also be given through other devices, e.g. 'turbuhaler' or 'nebuliser', which release a regulated dose.

CAUSES

Factors triggering an asthma attack include:

▶ exercise

▶ respiratory infections

▶ allergies (e.g. to pollens, foods, bee sting)

▶ exposure to a sudden change in weather conditions, especially cold air

▶ anxiety or emotional stress

▶ house dust

▶ smoke

▶ certain food additives or preservatives

MANAGEMENT OF AN ASTHMA ATTACK

1 Follow DRABC. **DRABC**

2 Assist the casualty, if conscious, into a comfortable position—usually sitting upright and leaning forward.

3 Be reassuring and ensure adequate fresh air.

4 Assist with prompt administration of medication:
- give 4 puffs of a blue reliever inhaler (puffer) containing Ventolin, Respolin, Respax, Asmol, or Bricanyl
- casualty takes a breath with each puff

• use a spacer if available: give 4 puffs one at a time—casualty takes 4 breaths after each puff—wait 4 minutes
• if no improvement, give another 4 puffs.

5 If little or no benefit:
☎ *call 000 for an ambulance.*

6 For a severe attack with little or no improvement, keep giving 4 puffs every 4 minutes until ambulance arrives:
- children 4 puffs each time is a safe dose
- adults up to 6–8 puffs every 5 minutes may be given for a severe attack while waiting for the ambulance.

7 **If casualty unconscious**, follow DRABC:
☎ *call 000 for an ambulance.*

Where permitted under local State or Territory regulations:

- ▶ use another person's reliever inhaler or use one from a first aid kit to assist a casualty with a severe asthma attack
- ▶ if someone is having difficulty breathing, but has not previously had an asthma attack, assist in giving 4 puffs of a reliever and continue with 4 puffs every 4 minutes if required until an ambulance arrives

LIVING WITH ASTHMA

Although it is treatable, there is no known cure for asthma. However, children tend to grow out of it.

Asthma can affect people differently. Recognising and treating symptoms early can reduce the severity of an attack.

ASSESSING THE SEVERITY OF AN ASTHMA ATTACK

Mild	*Moderate*	*Severe* *
• cough, soft wheeze	• persistent cough, loud wheeze	• very distressed, anxious
• minor difficulty breathing	• obvious difficulty breathing	• gasping for breath
• no difficulty speaking in sentences	• able to speak in short sentences only	• able to speak only a few gasping words in one breath
		• pale and sweaty
		• may have blue lips

WARNING: Anyone having a SEVERE asthma attack needs URGENT medical treatment.

☎ *Call 000 for an ambulance.*

Successful asthma management aims at prevention so that the person's lifestyle is unaffected. All asthmatics should develop an Asthma Management Plan with their own doctor.

EXERCISE-INDUCED ASTHMA

However some people may not have an Asthma Management Plan because they do not give management of their asthma high priority.

The majority of people who have asthma lead normal lives. Many take part in competitive sport. During exercise the airways dry out, due to an increased air intake, increasing susceptibility to an attack. There can be a great deal of variation from day to day in the occurrence and severity of asthma, although it is known that:

- an attack is more likely after prolonged strenuous running (e.g. a cross-country race)
- symptoms can occur soon after exercise (in cool-down period) as well as during activity

People with asthma should exercise to improve their general fitness and lung function. However, they should avoid exercise when:

- they have a viral infection
- symptoms of asthma are already apparent
- a known allergen (e.g. pollen) is present
- the air is unusually cold

Preventive measures can be taken by asthmatic sportspeople:

- use a reliever inhaler 5–10 minutes before exercise
- do a warm-up:
  - a 2–3 minute jog, followed by:
    a 30 second sprint, then 1 minute rest
    (repeat sprint/rest cycle 5–7 times)
    OR
  - a brisk walk or slow jog of 20–30 minutes
- do stretching exercises

CARE OF A PUFFER

- ▶ remove medication cylinder from inhaler
- ▶ wash plastic inhaler in warm, soapy water
- ▶ clear nozzle hole of residue (inside inhaler)
- ▶ rinse inhaler in clean water and air dry

CARE OF A SPACER

- ▶ remove puffer from spacer
- ▶ wash spacer in warm water with kitchen detergent
- ▶ drain and air dry–**do not** rinse
- ▶ **do not** use a cloth to dry spacer

EXTERNAL CLUES TO MEDICAL CONDITIONS

Casualties may have items with them which give vital clues about the emergency. Medical warning items (such as a Medic-Alert bracelet), a puffer, an EpiPen™, or other medicines carried on the person, can all be clues to what has caused the emergency.

ALLERGIES

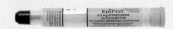

EpiPen™ (a self injector containing adrenaline) indicates a tendency to allergic reactions

ASTHMA
Puffer is often carried by people with asthma

DIABETES
Insulin injector or blood glucose meter are carried by diabetics. Sugar lumps or sweets may also indicate diabetes

Medic-Alert bracelet or similar gives information about medical condition

Medication—glyceryl trinitrate is taken for angina; phenytoin for epilepsy; indigestion or antacid tablets may indicate a stomach ulcer

DIABETES

Diabetes is caused by a disorder of the pancreas. In the digestive process, the body breaks foods down into sugars which are absorbed into the bloodstream. In a healthy person, the pancreas then produces insulin to convert this sugar into energy. In diabetes, insulin production and function are impaired. Sugar builds up in the blood, and the cells don't get the energy they need.

The term diabetes covers a range of closely related conditions including:
- insulin-dependent diabetes—thought to be caused by an auto-immune process which causes a loss of insulin production
- non-insulin dependent diabetes—thought to be associated with factors such as obesity, common in Western lifestyles
- impaired glucose tolerance—more common in obese people and thought to be an early stage of diabetes

Diabetics must carefully monitor diet and exercise, and may require regular insulin or other medication. A person suffering from diabetes may have a glucometer—battery powered instrument used to collect a drop of blood and measure the blood glucose level.

Diabetic emergencies A diabetic emergency may result from too much or too little insulin in the blood. There are two types of diabetic emergency—very low blood sugar (hypoglycaemia, usually due to excessive insulin); or very high blood sugar (hyperglycaemia, due to insufficient insulin).

The more common emergency is hypoglycaemia.
This can result from too much insulin or other
medication, not having eaten enough of the
correct food, unaccustomed exercise or a
missed meal.

Signs and symptoms   If caused by **low blood sugar**, the person may:
- feel dizzy, weak, trembly and hungry
- look pale and have a rapid pulse
- be sweating profusely
- be numb around lips and fingers
- appear confused or aggressive
- be unconscious

If caused by **high blood sugar**, the person may:
- be excessively thirsty
- have a frequent need to urinate
- have hot dry skin, a rapid pulse, drowsiness
- have the smell of acetone (like nail polish
  remover) on the breath
- be unconscious

*If unsure whether attack is caused by low or high
blood sugar, give a sweet (sugar-containing)
drink. Do not use 'diet' soft drinks. This could
save the person's life, if blood sugar is low, and
will not cause undue harm if blood sugar is high.*

Although you may not be able to determine the
type of diabetic emergency or be able to find out
from the casualty, it is important that you
recognise the casualty's condition as an
emergency and get medical aid quickly.

MANAGEMENT OF DIABETIC EMERGENCY

CAUSED BY LOW BLOOD SUGAR

If casualty unconscious:

1 Follow DRABC.

2 Give nothing by mouth.

3 ☎ *Call 000 for an ambulance.*

If casualty conscious:

1 Give sugar, glucose or a sweet drink (e.g. soft drink or cordial—do not use 'diet' soft drinks or diabetic-type cordials).

2 Continue giving sugar every 15 minutes until medical aid arrives or casualty recovers.

3 Loosen tight clothing.

4 Seek medical aid if required.

CAUSED BY HIGH BLOOD SUGAR

If casualty unconscious:

1 Follow DRABC. DRABC

2 Give nothing by mouth.

3 ☎ *Call 000 for an ambulance.*

If casualty conscious:

1 Allow casualty to self-administer insulin (do not administer it yourself, but help if needed).

A casualty who has diabetes may carry a NovoPen™ to inject insulin.

2 Seek medical aid if required. If help delayed, encourage casualty to drink sugar-free fluids.

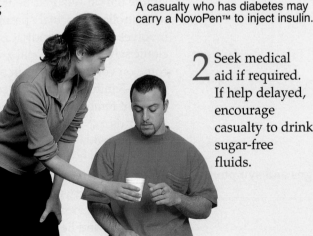

Epilepsy and Other Seizures

Epilepsy is a disorder of the nervous system characterised by seizures (convulsions, sometimes called 'fits'). A seizure is not necessarily the result of epilepsy but can be caused by a head injury, high fever, brain tumour, poisoning, drug overdose, stroke, infection, or anything which severely impairs supply of oxygen or blood to the brain.

One in every hundred Australians has a form of epilepsy. One in every twenty children will have an episode of febrile convulsions caused by high body temperature—*see Infantile Convulsions p. 189.* The management of seizures is the same irrespective of the cause. People with epilepsy may be aware that they are about to have a seizure because of a brief sensation—a perceived sound, a smell, or a feeling of movement. This is termed an 'aura'.

Seizures range from a mild blackout called a simple partial seizure ('petit mal') to sudden uncontrolled muscular spasms. If a seizure involves the whole body it is referred to as a tonic clonic seizure ('grand mal'). A major seizure can come on very suddenly but seldom lasts longer than 2–3 minutes. After the seizure the person may not remember what happened and may appear dazed and confused as well as sleepy or exhausted.

Signs and symptoms

A person having an epileptic seizure may:
- suddenly cry out
- fall to the ground (sometimes resulting in injury) and lie rigid for a few seconds
- have a congested and blue face and neck

▶ have jerky, spasmodic muscular movements
▶ froth at the mouth
▶ bite the tongue
▶ lose control of bladder and bowel

MANAGEMENT OF AN EPILEPTIC SEIZURE

During the convulsion

1 **DO NOT** try to restrain the person.

2 **DO NOT** put anything in the mouth.

3 Protect person from obvious injury.

4 Place something soft under head and shoulders.

After the convulsion

1 Follow DRABC. **DRABC**▶

2 Place on side in recovery position as soon as possible to keep airway clear.

3 Manage injuries resulting from seizure.

4 **DO NOT** disturb if casualty falls asleep but continue to check ABC.

Seek medical aid if:
- the seizure continues for more than 5 minutes
- another seizure quickly follows
- the person has been injured

ALLERGIC REACTIONS

An allergic reaction can occur when a substance enters the body. The allergy may be to an insect sting or bite, drugs, medication, food or chemicals.

An allergic reaction may be potentially fatal and therefore need urgent medical attention. Such a serious reaction may cause blood pressure to fall dramatically and breathing to be impaired (anaphylactic shock). The face and neck can become swollen, increasing the risk of suffocation, and the amount of oxygen reaching the vital organs (heart, lungs and brain) may be severely reduced *(see p.328)*.

Signs and symptoms

▶ swelling and redness of the skin
▶ itchy, raised rash (hives)
▶ swelling of the throat
▶ wheezing and/or coughing
▶ rapid, irregular pulse
▶ nausea and vomiting
▶ dizziness or unconsciousness

MANAGEMENT OF SEVERE ALLERGIC REACTION

1 Follow DRABC.

2 ☎ *Call 000 for an ambulance.*

3 Observe and record pulse and breathing.

4 If the casualty is carrying medication for the allergy, it should be taken at once.

5 **If conscious:** help casualty to sit in position that most relieves breathing difficulty.

If unconscious: check ABC and prepare to resuscitate if necessary.

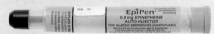

Some people are aware of their hypersensitivity, so check (e.g. in a handbag) for a syringe of adrenaline (EpiPen™). Assist casualty to use it.

INFANTILE CONVULSIONS

A rapid rise in temperature, to even as little as 38.5°C (normal is 37°C), can cause convulsions in infants and young children, most often those aged 10 months to 5 years. This high temperature or fever is usually caused by a cold or other viral illness. Infantile convulsions are usually brief, lasting no more than 5 minutes, and are quite common.

Note: Convulsions caused by high temperature—called febrile convulsions—can also occur in adults.

Signs and symptoms

▶ fever
▶ twitching of face or limbs
▶ eyes rolling up
▶ congestion of face and neck
▶ blue face and lips
▶ stiffness of body with arched back
▶ unconsciousness

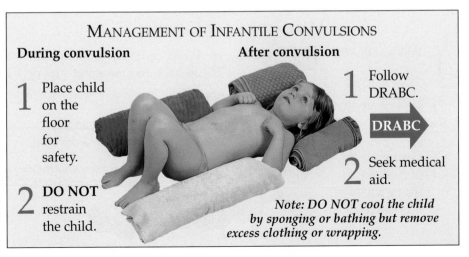

MANAGEMENT OF INFANTILE CONVULSIONS

During convulsion

1 Place child on the floor for safety.

2 **DO NOT** restrain the child.

After convulsion

1 Follow DRABC.

DRABC▶

2 Seek medical aid.

Note: DO NOT cool the child by sponging or bathing but remove excess clothing or wrapping.

189

FAINTING

Fainting is a partial or complete loss of consciousness caused by a temporary reduction of blood flow to the brain. It can be triggered by emotional shock, pain, over-exertion, exhaustion, lack of food, sight of blood or, in most cases, standing immobile in hot conditions. Some people, such as pregnant women or the elderly, can faint as a result of changing position (e.g. from sitting to standing). But fainting can occur at any time. It results in a brief loss of consciousness, slow pulse and pallor.

Signs and symptoms

The casualty may feel light-headed, dizzy, or nauseated, and have a pale, cool, moist skin and numbness in the fingers and toes.

Usually people recover quickly, often within seconds, without any lasting effects. If fainting is the result of an underlying medical condition, however, the casualty should see a doctor.

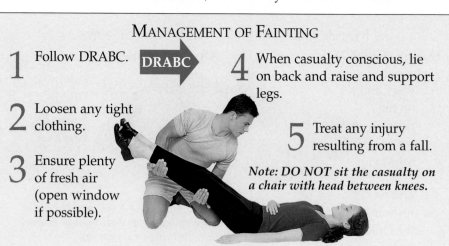

MANAGEMENT OF FAINTING

1 Follow DRABC. **DRABC**

2 Loosen any tight clothing.

3 Ensure plenty of fresh air (open window if possible).

4 When casualty conscious, lie on back and raise and support legs.

5 Treat any injury resulting from a fall.

Note: DO NOT sit the casualty on a chair with head between knees.

11

Exposure to heat and cold

One tenth of Australia has significant periods of below freezing weather, and most of the continent has extensive periods of extreme heat. Australians travel overseas to areas where they may experience extremes of temperature. Exposure to these extremes of heat or cold may cause suffering, injury, and even death.

These situations are not confined to the outback or snowfields. The casualty may be the elderly person sitting quietly in a cold room, the homeless teenager wandering the streets, the victim of a boating mishap, the lost bushwalker or even the person exercising in the middle of a hot summer's day.

This chapter discusses what first aid can be given to casualties suffering from conditions caused by heat and cold, and also focuses on prevention.

EXPOSURE TO HEAT AND COLD

The body works efficiently only as long as it remains at a constant temperature. If the body's temperature drops more than a few degrees below the normal of approximately 37°C, or rises significantly, it cannot function properly.

MAINTAINING NORMAL BODY TEMPERATURE

The body is like a house with an efficient ducted heating and cooling system. It maintains a constant temperature by balancing heat production and heat loss.

Sources of heat

Eating provides the body with fuel to burn. The conversion of food into energy (the process of metabolism) provides much of the body's heat as does muscular activity such as exercising or shivering. Heat is also absorbed from outside sources such as the sun, hot air or hot food.

Cooling

The circulatory system provides the ducting system. When the body needs to lose heat, blood vessels near the surface of the skin widen (dilate) to allow more warm blood to be brought to the skin's surface for heat to escape. The evaporation of sweat from the skin's surface also causes heat loss.

Moving air—from a fan or a breeze—speeds up the cooling process. The faster air moves, the quicker sweat evaporates and the layer of warmed air around the body is swept away.

Conserving heat

If the body needs to conserve heat, blood vessels near the skin's surface get smaller (constrict) to keep heat inside. The skin looks pale or white and feels cold. Sweating stops and muscles contract causing goose bumps which raise hairs on the body in an attempt to 'trap' warm air at the skin's surface.

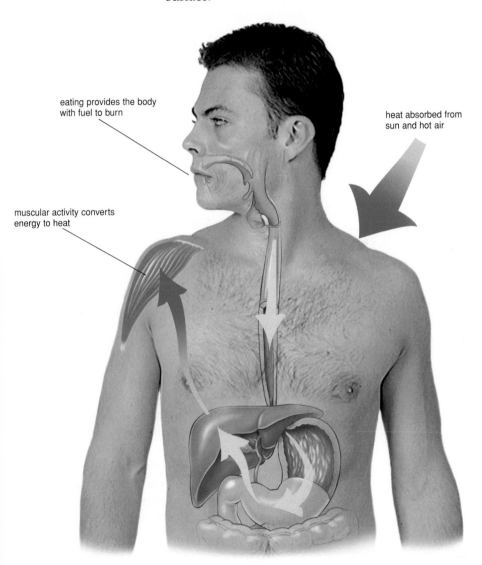

eating provides the body with fuel to burn

heat absorbed from sun and hot air

muscular activity converts energy to heat

THE HOT ENVIRONMENT

People are at risk of heat illness in humid or hot climates. Someone working in a hot environment, such as a boiler room, is at risk because the air heats the body at a rate faster than it can cool itself.

In a hot, dry climate, evaporation is very fast; therefore the body can adapt to the higher temperatures. In a humid climate, evaporation is slower. It can be more difficult to maintain core body temperature in Cairns when it is 25°C and humid than in Bourke at a dry 35°C.

The importance of water

Heat can interfere with the body's water balance. The body needs a minimum amount of water to carry out normal functions such as blood circulation and excretion of waste. For healthy adults in non-active, cool conditions, a minimum water intake of about 1.7 litres per day is needed. In hot climates, where physical work is being undertaken in the open, an intake of up to 15 litres per day may be required.

Heavy sweating removes water and salts from the body at a faster rate than normal. Total blood volume decreases because there is less fluid available for the plasma. More salt and water are retained by the kidneys. Collection of urine in the bladder is slower, with a higher concentration of waste products causing urine to be a darker yellow colour. This is a warning sign that plasma volume is falling. If this is not corrected, the body becomes dehydrated.

People do not always realise they are not replacing fluid being lost through sweating. They may not feel thirsty—or thirsty enough—to realise the importance of drinking more water. Because of this, troops on training exercises and people in fun runs or working out at gyms are taught and encouraged to drink water at regular intervals.

When moving to a hot climate, one needs to increase daily intake of water. Body salts may also be depleted, so extra salt may be needed in food. If water is replaced but not body salts, the concentration of salt will be too low, impairing normal functioning. With time—within 2 weeks, adaptation decreases the amount of water and salt lost.

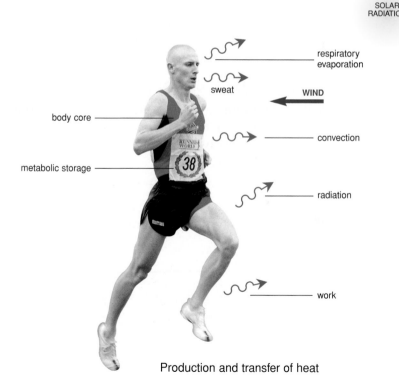

Production and transfer of heat

HEAT-INDUCED CONDITIONS

Physical activity, particularly in hot conditions, can result in the body becoming overheated. This can result in:

▶ **heat-induced swelling**—feet and hands swell in warm weather

MANAGEMENT

1 Raise legs.

2 Do gentle exercise.

3 Keep cool.

▶ **heat cramps**—painful muscle cramps, usually in legs and abdomen, caused by losing too much water and salt through sweating

MANAGEMENT

1 Stop the activity and rest in a cool environment.

2 Gently stretch the affected muscle.

3 Apply an ice pack.

4 Replace fluids.

In addition to swelling and cramps, more serious heat-induced conditions can also develop.

HEAT EXHAUSTION

Heat exhaustion results from being physically active in a hot environment, without taking the right precautions. It can affect athletes, workers who must wear heavy clothing (e.g. firefighters, factory workers), the young, the elderly who compensate poorly for heat, those wearing unsuitable clothing on a hot day, and people suffering from dehydration.

Fluid loss through sweating reduces the amount of water in the body so that the blood volume falls. Increasing blood flow to the skin makes the blood volume even less effective, reducing blood flow to vital organs. As the circulatory system is affected, the body goes into a mild form of shock.

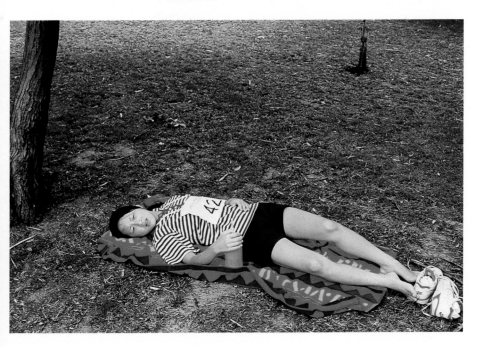

Signs and symptoms

- feeling hot, exhausted and weak
- persistent headache
- thirst and nausea
- giddiness and faintness
- fatigue
- rapid breathing and shortness of breath
- pale, cool, clammy skin
- rapid, weak pulse

MANAGEMENT OF HEAT EXHAUSTION

1 Move casualty to lie down in a cool place with circulating air.

2 Loosen tight clothing and remove unnecessary garments.

3 Sponge with cold water.

4 Give fluids to drink.

5 Seek medical aid if casualty vomits or does not recover promptly.

HEATSTROKE

Heatstroke is a potentially lethal condition. Water levels in the body become so low that sweating stops and body temperature rises because the body can no longer cool itself. The brain and other vital organs, such as the kidneys and heart, begin to fail.

Those most at risk of heatstroke include infants left in closed cars on a warm to hot day, athletes attempting to run long distances in hot weather, unfit workers and overweight alcoholics in hot climates, the elderly and the sick.

Signs and symptoms

▶ high body temperature of 40°C or more
▶ flushed, dry skin
▶ initially a pounding, rapid pulse which gradually weakens
▶ headache, nausea and/or vomiting
▶ dizziness and visual disturbances
▶ irritability and mental confusion
▶ altered mental state which may progress to seizures and unconsciousness

MANAGEMENT OF HEATSTROKE

1 Follow DRABC. **DRABC▶**

2 Remove casualty to a cool place.

3 Remove almost all clothing; loosen anything tight.

4 Apply cold packs or ice to areas of large blood vessels (neck, groin and armpits) to accelerate cooling.

5 If possible, cover body with a wet sheet; fan to increase air circulation (stop cooling when body cold to the touch).

6 ☎ *Call 000 for an ambulance.*

7 When casualty fully conscious, give fluids.

THE COLD ENVIRONMENT

MAINTAINING BODY TEMPERATURE

Just as the body reacts to external heat conditions, it also reacts to cold. To conserve body heat, blood vessels in the skin shut down to prevent the body's 'core heat' escaping. This will affect extremities (fingers and toes) before other exposed areas of the body.

Wind and skin wetness increase the effects of cold air. Wind speed and air temperature combine to give the 'windchill factor'.

Clothing, food and water intake, and physical exercise can also affect body cooling.

Windchill nomogram
The red line shows an example of an air temperature of –20°C and a wind speed of 8 metres per second being equivalent to a temperature of –32°C on exposed flesh.

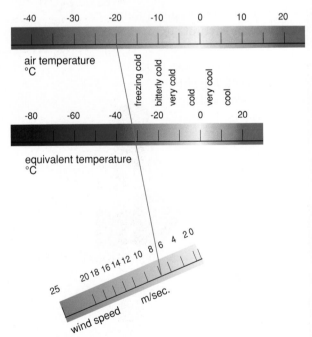

HOW THE BODY LOSES HEAT

Heat may be lost by

▶ **radiation**
  • heat radiates from the body, especially from the head

▶ **evaporation**
  • the body produces sweat which evaporates from the skin's surface to keep the body cool on a hot day
  • breathing: cold air is inhaled, warmed and humidified by the body, and exhaled—the moisture in exhaled air, on a cold day, condenses into a misty breath

▶ **conduction**
  • when you sit on or touch a cold object, heat flows directly from the body to the cold surface (e.g. sitting on a cold chair or the cold ground)

▶ **convection**
  • the thin layer of air on the surface of the skin rises and is replaced by cooler air, causing heat loss (even in the absence of wind or movement)

How the body loses heat

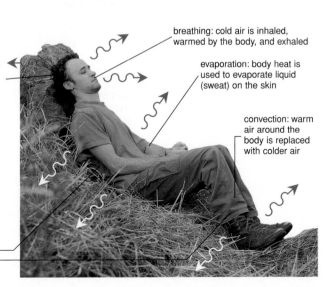

radiation from the body, especially the head, into the air around it

breathing: cold air is inhaled, warmed by the body, and exhaled

evaporation: body heat is used to evaporate liquid (sweat) on the skin

convection: warm air around the body is replaced with colder air

conduction: heat moves from the warm body to a cold object that the body is in contact with

Humans are able to adjust to the cold in a number of ways:

By decreasing heat loss:

▶ exposure to cold conditions causes blood vessels near skin surface to constrict, thereby reducing the amount of heat radiated away

▶ use of clothing and shelter insulates the body from cold and wind

▶ use of artificial heating warms the surroundings—decreasing the difference between ambient and body temperatures

By increasing heat production:

▶ exercise causes metabolic heat production to increase considerably

▶ shivering is a form of involuntary exercise which occurs as the core temperature starts to drop

People most at risk

Anyone can suffer cold-induced conditions related to over-exposure. Some groups are particularly prone. They include:

▶ the elderly—often have poor circulation, reduced body insulation and low metabolic rate

▶ babies and young children—lose body heat quickly, especially from head

▶ people already weakened through lack of food, fatigue or injury

▶ people under the influence of alcohol or other drugs—more because of effect on behaviour than any possible alcohol-induced dilation of the blood vessels

▶ those with certain health problems—e.g. thyroid and pituitary disorders, trauma, burns, starvation, strokes, certain skin conditions, those confined to bed or a wheelchair, and those taking certain medication (especially some psychiatric drugs)

▶ anyone who is trapped or immobilised

COLD-INDUCED CONDITIONS

Signs and symptoms

When body temperature falls, early warning signs may include:
- feeling cold
- shivering
- clumsiness and slurred speech
- apathy and irrational behaviour

As the body temperature continues to drop:
- shivering usually ceases
- pulse may be difficult to find
- heart rate may slow
- level of consciousness continues to decline

Around 30°C body temperature:
- unconsciousness is likely
- heart rhythm is increasingly likely to change

As the body temperature falls further the heart may arrest, resulting in death.

HYPOTHERMIA

Hypothermia occurs when the body's warming mechanisms fail or are overwhelmed and body temperature drops below 35°C. Hypothermia has the potential to develop into a serious condition if not recognised and treated at an early stage.

Sometimes hypothermia is mistaken for other conditions such as drunkenness, a stroke or drug abuse. This is especially so in a city where it might be assumed that conditions would be unlikely to cause hypothermia.

MANAGEMENT OF HYPOTHERMIA

1 Follow DRABC. **DRABC**

2 Remove casualty to a warm, dry place.

3 Protect casualty and yourself from wind, rain, sleet, cold, and wet ground.

4 Handle casualty as gently as possible.

5 Avoid excess activity or movement.

6 Maintain casualty in a horizontal position.

7 Remove wet clothing.

8 Place casualty between blankets or in sleeping bag, and wrap in a space blanket * or similar.

9 Cover the head to maintain body heat.

* Note: Although a space blanket reflects radiated heat back to the body, it can also conduct heat away unless some form of insulation (blankets, sleeping mat, even thick layers of newspaper) is provided, either inside or outside the space blanket.

10 Give warm drinks if conscious (but not alcohol).

11 Provide warmth to the casualty—
• direct body-to-body contact is fairly ineffective and may even interfere with casualty's spontaneous rewarming by shivering; however, it may be the only means of rewarming available
• hot water bottles, heat packs and other sources of external heating may be applied to casualty's neck, armpits and groin, but caution must be taken to avoid burns; aim to stabilise core temperature rather than attempt rapid rewarming.

12 If hypothermia is severe:
☎ *call 000 for an ambulance.*

13 Remain with casualty until medical aid arrives.

Always consider the possibility of hypothermia if the weather is cold and wet or windy, and especially if all three conditions apply; following immersion; in those inadequately clothed; and in 'at risk' groups such as infants or the elderly.

Babies may also become hypothermic in rooms which would not pose a threat to an adult. Babies lose heat very easily. A baby may look healthy, the only signs of hypothermia being cold skin and that the baby is unusually quiet and drowsy or refuses food.

Cautions in first aid for hypothermia

▶ pulse may be difficult to find; check with a warm hand for 30 to 45 seconds
▶ if casualty starts to shiver, take measures to prevent further heat loss
▶ **DO NOT** rub affected area
▶ **DO NOT** use radiant heat such as fire or electric heaters
▶ **DO NOT** give alcohol

Note: It is best not to put casualty in a hot bath, as monitoring and/or resuscitation, if needed, may be difficult.

FROSTBITE

Frostbite occurs when the skin and underlying tissues become frozen as a result of exposure to below zero temperatures. It is a progressive injury. In **superficial frostbite** the skin can still be moved in relation to the underlying tissue. The full thickness of the skin is frozen. When only the top layer of the skin is frozen, the condition is sometimes referred to as frostnip. **Deep frostbite** is recognisable by the skin no longer being mobile in relation to the underlying tissue. The skin and the tissues underneath the skin are frozen, sometimes to the bone.

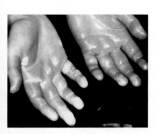

Frostbitten fingers before thawing

Stages of frostbite

Stage	Description	Signs and symptoms
superficial frostbite	The full thickness of the skin is frozen. If only the top layer of the skin is frozen, it is usually called frostnip.	• white, waxy-looking skin • skin is firm to touch, but tissue underneath is soft • may feel pain at first, followed by numbness
deep frostbite	The skin, and the tissues underneath the skin, are frozen, sometimes to the bone. A serious condition, often involving an entire hand or foot.	• white, waxy-looking skin that turns greyish-blue as frostbite progresses • skin feels cold and hard • there is no feeling in the area

DO NOT rub or massage the frozen area—the tiny ice crystals in the tissues may cause more tissue damage.

DO NOT rewarm with radiant heat (fire, exhaust pipes)—this may rewarm too quickly.

DO NOT apply snow or cold water to area—this may cause further freezing and tissue damage.

DO NOT give person alcohol.

CRYOGENIC BURN

A cryogenic burn occurs when the skin touches and sticks to an extremely cold surface, such as metal or ice, or comes into contact with liquefied gases, resulting in frostbite. Wearing gloves can prevent this.

MANAGEMENT OF SUPERFICIAL FROSTBITE

1 Follow DRABC. **DRABC**

2 Remove casualty to a warm, dry place.

3 Rewarm the frostbitten part with body heat (e.g. place frostbitten fingers in armpit, place warm hands over frost-bitten ears).

4 Prevent affected areas from freezing by ensuring that casualty stops the activity or dresses more appropriately.

MANAGEMENT OF DEEP FROSTBITE

1 Follow DRABC.

2 Prevent further heat loss from the frozen part and the rest of the body.

3 Handle the frozen tissue very gently to prevent further tissue damage.

4 **DO NOT** rub the arms and legs; keep the casualty as still as possible.

5 Remove casualty to a warm, dry place—if the feet or legs are frozen, don't let the casualty walk.

6 ☎ *Call 000 for an ambulance.*

If medical help not readily available, thaw the frozen part as follows:

1 Make the casualty warm and as comfortable as possible.

2 Gently remove the clothing from affected part.

3 Fill a container, large enough to hold the entire frozen part, with warm water (about 40°C—feels warm to the elbow).

4 Remove any jewellery; put the whole frozen part in the water.

5 Keep adding warm water to maintain a constant temperature.

6 Keep the part in the water until it is pink or does not improve any more—this can take up to 40 minutes, and may be painful.

7 Keep the part elevated and warm; do not break any blisters that form.

8 ☎ *Call 000 for an ambulance.*

MANAGEMENT OF CRYOGENIC BURN

1 Pour warm water over the part to free it.

2 When free, treat as for superficial frostbite.

3 Seek medical aid for blistering or other tissue damage.

FOCUS ON SAFETY

Preventing heat-induced conditions

- avoid being outside in the part of the day when radiant heat is highest
- avoid strenuous exercise during hottest part of day; exercise in the cool of early morning or evening
- take frequent breaks in the shade to allow body to readjust temperature
- drink fluids at regular intervals
- do not wear too many layers of clothing in hot weather; wear light coloured clothes of natural fibres; cover body with light clothing to prevent sunburn and provide insulation from radiant heat; wear a hat

Preventing cold-induced conditions

- dress for weather and activity—in cold weather, prepare for rain or snow; wear waterproof and windproof outer clothing with wool or high insulation synthetic fibre underneath; dress in layers to trap warm air, and to allow you to take off layers if necessary, to avoid sweating; wear warm head covering and gloves or mittens
- keep dry—being wet, from rain or sweating, causes heat loss; take shelter before it rains; stop physical activity before sweating dampens your clothing, or adjust layers
- act safely—do not stay out for a long time or go on long walks when weather conditions are extreme; do not go out alone
- emergency food—ensure adequate hydration and nutrition; seek specialist advice on what is appropriate for your planned activity
- exercise—if you start to feel cold, movement will generate more heat (e.g. jogging, knee bends and arm swinging); if a significant degree of hypothermia is already present, do not force too much exercise or long walk to shelter
- in sub-freezing environment, watch each other for white noses and ears to prevent frostnip becoming frostbite

Burns and scalds

Burns can be extremely painful. Risk of infection is high because the outer layer of skin is broken. Although they do not bleed, burns can result in fluid loss, loss of temperature control and can damage underlying layers of tissue and nerves. If extensive, burns may also damage the respiratory system and eyes, and the casualty may go into shock.

As well as obvious physical damage, burns can also cause psychological damage as they can be disfiguring and disabling.

Burns are primarily caused by dry heat (e.g. flames, a hot object), but can also be caused by extreme cold, chemicals, electricity, or the sun and other forms of radiation. Even after the source of heat has been removed, there can be further damage because soft tissue retains heat for minutes afterwards.

Cooling the burnt area and preventing infection are the first aider's major objectives. In some cases, the first aider will also have to ensure the casualty does not go into respiratory or cardiac arrest, or shock.

BURNS AND SCALDS

Burns are injuries to the skin and underlying tissues caused by heat, extreme cold, chemicals, corrosive substances, electricity, friction (e.g. rope burn) and radiation (e.g. the sun, microwaves, snow, sun lamps). Scalds are burns caused by hot liquid and steam.

Children under five and the elderly are more at risk because their skin is thinner. People who have heart conditions, kidney problems or chronic illnesses, or who are malnourished, are also at greater risk.

THE SEVERITY OF A BURN

The severity of a burn depends on:
▶   extent of burn
▶   part(s) of body burnt
▶   depth of burn
▶   age and physical condition of casualty

The extent and depth of burns can be influenced by the temperature of the object, liquid or gas that caused the burn, and the length of time the casualty was exposed to burning.

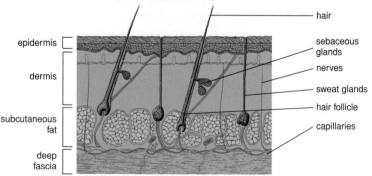

epidermis

dermis

subcutaneous fat

deep fascia

hair

sebaceous glands

nerves

sweat glands

hair follicle

capillaries

Superficial burns

In a superficial burn, only the top layer (epidermis) of the skin is damaged. A common example is radiation by ultraviolet light producing sunburn. If severe, some fluid may leak into the epidermis causing swelling and blistering.

Superficial partial thickness burns

Superficial partial thickness burns occur when the upper layers of the dermis are injured resulting in leakage of fluid into the tissues, producing blistering. These burns are commonly caused by brief exposure to flame or spill scalds of 50–70°C. The area is red or mottled red and white, very painful and blistered with copious tissue fluids.

epidermis

dermis

subcutaneous fat

deep fascia

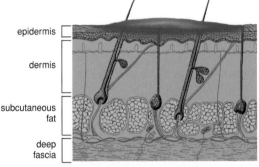 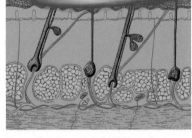

Superficial burn (sunburn)   Superficial partial thickness burn

Deep partial thickness burns

Deep partial thickness burns involve the epidermis and much of the dermis. They are caused by scalds of longer duration or temperature of more than 70°C, or exposure to flame. The area is dark red or pale yellow, denuded of epidermis, with a moist surface.

Full thickness burns

Full thickness burns involve the epidermis and the entire dermis. They may be caused by flame burns, contact with hot metal, immersion scalds, strong chemicals or electricity. The area is white or charred and feels dry and leathery. Because the nerves are destroyed, the pain may not be as great as in a less severe burn.

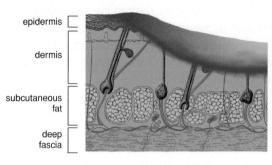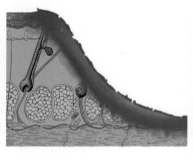

epidermis

dermis

subcutaneous fat

deep fascia

Deep (dermal) partial thickness burn   Full thickness burn

Critical burns

Some burns are classed as critical and include:

▶ burns that interfere with breathing
▶ burns where there is serious soft tissue injury or fracture
▶ burns to the face, feet, genitals, neck, knees, elbows and other areas where the skin folds
▶ all electrical burns
▶ most chemical burns
▶ burns to young children and people over 50 years old
▶ burns to people with serious medical conditions such as diabetes, seizure disorders, hypertension, respiratory difficulties or mental illness

---

GENERAL PRINCIPLES FOR MANAGING BURNS

1 Follow DRABC.   (or aluminium foil, plastic wrap, or a wet clean dressing).

2 Cool the burnt area.

3 Cover the burnt area with a non-adherent/burns dressing

4 Prevent infection.

5 Minimise shock.

COMPLICATIONS FROM BURNS

Severe burns

Burn injuries can affect more than just the burnt tissue. Severe burns also impact on the major body systems. Complications include:

- shock caused by loss of blood or blood plasma
- infection (the deeper the burn, the higher the risk)
- breathing problems if face and/or throat is burnt or casualty has inhaled smoke, gas or fumes
- circulation restricted or cut off by swelling

DO NOT apply lotions, ointments or oily dressings.

DO NOT prick or break blisters.

DO NOT give alcohol.

DO NOT overcool casualty (particularly if young or if burn extensive).

DO NOT use towels, cotton wool, blankets or adhesive dressings directly on wound.

DO NOT remove clothing stuck to burnt area.

WHEN TO SEEK MEDICAL AID

Extensive burns

Extensive burns are dangerous and may be fatal. Seek medical aid if:

- burn is deep, even if casualty does not feel any pain
- a superficial burn is larger than a 20 cent piece
- the burn involves airway, hands, face or genitals
- you are unsure of severity of burn

TYPES OF BURNS

THERMAL BURNS AND SCALDS

Thermal burns are those caused by heat—contact with an open flame or a hot object; scalding by steam or hot liquid; or burning by friction.

MANAGEMENT OF THERMAL BURNS

1 Follow DRABC.

2 Extinguish burning clothing—smother with blanket, jacket or use water (if a scald, quickly remove casualty's wet clothing from affected area).

3 Hold burnt area under cold, running water until it returns to normal temperature (up to 10 minutes).

4 Remove jewellery and clothing from burnt area (unless stuck).

5 Cover burn with a non-adherent/burns dressing (or aluminium foil, plastic wrap, or a wet clean dressing).

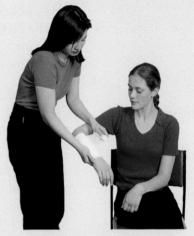

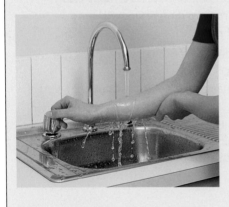

6 Seek medical aid urgently.

CLOTHES ON FIRE

If a person's clothes catch alight, it is vital to stop oxygen feeding the fire. Stop the person moving or running around as this will fan the flames. *Remember: STOP—DROP—ROLL—MANAGE.* **If your own clothes catch fire**, extinguish the flames by tightly wrapping a woollen blanket, coat or other suitable material around yourself and rolling along the ground. If no suitable material readily available, don't run around to find material: *STOP—DROP—ROLL.*

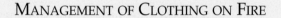

MANAGEMENT OF CLOTHING ON FIRE

1 **STOP** casualty running around.

2 **DROP** casualty to the ground and wrap in a blanket, coat or rug (wool is best; don't use anything made of nylon or other synthetic materials).

3 **ROLL** casualty along the ground until flames are smothered.

4 **MANAGE** as for a thermal burn.

5 Seek medical aid.

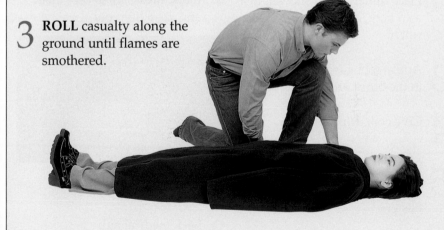

RADIATION BURNS

Radiation burns are caused by radiant energy—energy that radiates from its source. Sunburn is the most common. Radiation burns can also be caused by x-rays, welding equipment, and radioactive material.

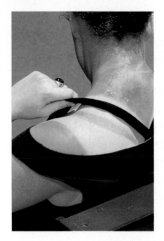

Sunburn is caused by overexposure to the sun (even on an overcast day). Some medication can make a person more prone to sunburn. Most sunburn is superficial but in severe cases, the skin may be 'lobster-red' and blistered.

If the eyes are burnt by the sun, they may feel gritty, painful and be sensitive to light.

MANAGEMENT OF SUNBURN

1 Rest casualty in a cool place.

2 Place under a cold shower, in a cold bath, or sponge with cold water.

3 Apply cool gauze padding to the burnt area.

4 Give cool drinks.

5 Seek medical aid for young babies and casualties with blisters.

Sunburn to eyes:

1 Cover eyes with thick, cool, moist dressings to cool them and keep light out.

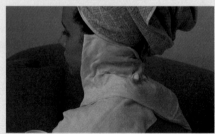

2 Reassure casualty.

3 Seek medical aid.

ELECTRICAL BURNS

An electrical burn may be more serious than it appears. It can be quite deep even when the surface skin shows no evidence of burning. High current flow can cause entry and exit wounds where the current density is highest, but most of the damage is to the deep tissues which can be severely damaged by heat. Current flow through the heart, especially alternating current (AC), may cause a cardiac arrest.

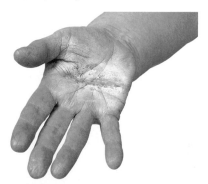

MANAGEMENT OF ELECTRICAL BURNS

1 Check for danger for yourself and bystanders.

2 Switch off power if possible.

3 Remove casualty from electrical supply without directly touching the casualty, using non-conductive, dry materials, e.g. dry wooden broom handle.

4 Follow DRABC.

5 Wash and cool burnt area under running water.

6 Apply a non-adherent/burns dressing (or aluminium foil, plastic wrap, or wet clean dressing).

7 ☎ *Call 000 for an ambulance.*

Note: If casualty is in contact with high voltage lines, do not approach but wait until power is disconnected by electricity authority personnel.

CHEMICAL BURNS

Burns are often caused by chemicals used in industry but can also result from chemical agents used in the home. Cleaning solutions (e.g. dish-washing powder, bleach and toilet bowl cleaners), paint strippers, and garden chemicals often contain caustic chemicals which can burn tissues.

A caustic chemical will continue to burn while in contact with the skin. Therefore it is very important to remove the chemical from the skin as quickly as possible.

Chemical burns to the eyes can cause permanent damage. The casualty may suffer extreme pain and be very sensitive to light *(see Eye Injuries, p. 165)*.

MANAGEMENT OF CHEMICAL BURNS

1   Follow DRABC.

2   **If chemical is on skin:**
- wash chemical off immediately—use large quantity of water for at least 20 minutes
- remove contaminated clothing and footwear (**avoid contaminating yourself**)
- do not pick off contaminants that stick to the skin.

If chemical is in the eye:
- tilt head back and turn to side

- protect uninjured eye
- gently flush injured eye with cool water for at least 20 minutes (keep eye open with fingers if necessary).

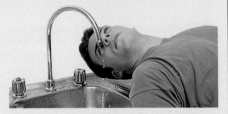

3   Cover area of eye with sterile or clean non-adherent dressing.

4   ☎ *Call 000 for an ambulance.*

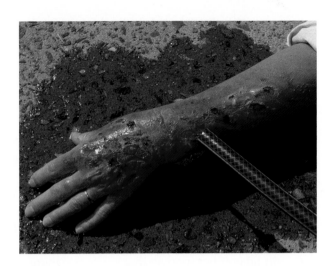

Chemical burn on arm
being washed with water

BITUMEN BURNS

Bitumen burns are normally caused through contact with or splashing of hot bitumen. It is important that the bitumen not be removed from the skin unless it is obstructing the airway, or further damage may result.

MANAGEMENT OF BITUMEN BURNS

1 Follow DRABC.

2 **DO NOT attempt to remove bitumen from skin or eyes.**

3 Drench burnt area immediately with cold, running water.

4 Apply cold, wet towels frequently.

5 Continue the cooling for 30 minutes **but no longer.**

6 If burn is to eye, flush eye with water for 20 minutes then cover the eye.

7 ☎ *Call 000 for an ambulance.*

Focus on Safety

Preventing thermal burns
- set thermostat on water heater around 50°C or fit a thermostatic control valve to water heater
- when preparing a bath, run cold water first, add hot water to required temperature, finish with cold water to cool taps
- keep hot liquids out-of-reach of children
- lift lids off hot food so that steam escapes away from you
- teach children the dangers of stoves, ovens, fireplaces, hot water taps, candles and matches
- turn saucepan handles away from edge of stove and out-of-reach of children
- don't leave young children alone in kitchen or bathroom
- buy only non-flammable clothing for children
- have guards on heaters and open fireplaces
- supervise use of stoves, fires, matches and lighters by young people

Preventing chemical burns
- wear eye protection when working with chemicals

- store chemicals out-of-reach of children and in a locked cupboard
- store chemicals low down, to guard against tipping when removing from storage

Preventing electrical burns
- secure electrical cords out-of-reach of children
- turn power points off and, if there are young children, fit child-proof dummy plugs
- turn electricity off and disconnect electrical equipment before repairing
- do not put knives and other metal objects into toasters
- check electrical cords for exposed wiring or broken covering
- consider installing earth leakage detectors in the home

Preventing radiation burns
- use protective clothing and sunscreen lotions (at least 15+)
- wear sunglasses
- be aware of medication which make your skin more sensitive to the sun

13

Poisoning

CONTENTS

The number of deaths in Australia from accidental poisonings has declined in recent years because of education campaigns and the introduction of child-proof containers. However, many thousands of accidental poisonings still occur, especially to children. People still lose their lives through poisoning.

Poisons can be ingested, inhaled, absorbed or injected into the body. Everyone is aware that Australia has a number of potentially lethal venomous snakes and spiders, and that poisonous fumes can be inhaled from a car exhaust or other toxic substance. However, many are not aware that some substances used in the home—cleaning products, pesticides, alcohol and medication—can also cause poisoning.

This chapter discusses sources of poisoning and how to manage its different forms.

POISONING

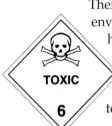

There are many substances in our immediate environment that are poisonous and, while some have a poisons symbol to indicate the danger, others do not. A **poison** is any substance which harms body tissues. A **toxin** is a poison made by an organism. A **venom** is a toxin injected by a fang or sting.

Tobacco, alcohol, some common plants, solvents, contaminated food, detergents, glues, adhesives, aerosols, and medication can be poisonous. Whether or not a substance is poisonous depends on the quantity taken in and, sometimes, on how it is absorbed. Many substances not harmful in small amounts can be poisonous in large amounts.

In every household there are caustic or petroleum substances which, if swallowed, can cause internal burns.

Poisoning can also occur in the workplace when workers are not aware of hazards associated with chemicals or are not fully acquainted with a task and necessary precautions.

Poisoning can be accidental or, rarely, intentional. Poisoning can result in permanent injury and death. Deaths occur from poisoning by household products, motor vehicle fumes, and chemicals used in hobbies, agriculture and industry. Poisoning can also result from the injection of venom from some creatures *(see ch. 14)*.

POISONS INFORMATION CENTRES

Poisons Information Centres exist in every State and Territory. The national number for information about poisons, and help in an emergency, is:

13 11 26

HOW POISONS ENTER THE BODY

Poisons can enter the body through the mouth (ingested/swallowed), nose (inhaled/breathed in) or skin (absorbed or injected). Once in the body, poisons may move into the bloodstream and be swiftly carried to all parts of the body.

HOW POISONS ENTER THE BODY

HOW POISONS AFFECT THE BODY

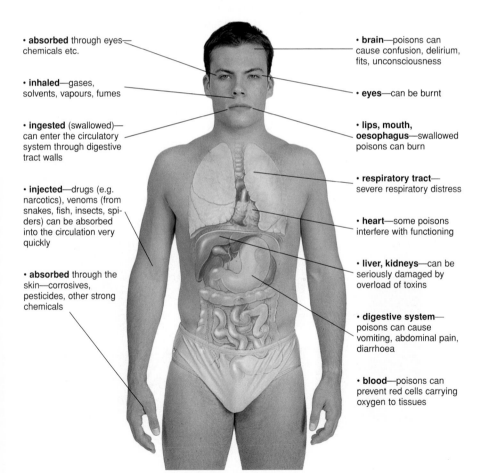

• **absorbed** through eyes—chemicals etc.

• **inhaled**—gases, solvents, vapours, fumes

• **ingested** (swallowed)—can enter the circulatory system through digestive tract walls

• **injected**—drugs (e.g. narcotics), venoms (from snakes, fish, insects, spiders) can be absorbed into the circulation very quickly

• **absorbed** through the skin—corrosives, pesticides, other strong chemicals

• **brain**—poisons can cause confusion, delirium, fits, unconsciousness

• **eyes**—can be burnt

• **lips, mouth, oesophagus**—swallowed poisons can burn

• **respiratory tract**—severe respiratory distress

• **heart**—some poisons interfere with functioning

• **liver, kidneys**—can be seriously damaged by overload of toxins

• **digestive system**—poisons can cause vomiting, abdominal pain, diarrhoea

• **blood**—poisons can prevent red cells carrying oxygen to tissues

INGESTED POISONS

Ingested poisons include contaminated or poisonous food (e.g. some mushrooms), substances such as alcohol, medication (e.g. paracetamol, tranquillisers—if taken in excess of normal dosage), household items (e.g. cleaners, dishwashing powders, kerosene, pesticides) and some plants (e.g. oleander).

Food poisoning, usually associated with poor hygiene and food handling, results from eating food contaminated by bacteria or by toxins produced by bacteria in the food at some stage. Bacterial food poisoning is often caused by *Salmonella* bacteria or by toxins from *Staphylococcus* bacteria.

Drinking large quantities of alcohol can result in poisoning. Alcohol depresses the activity of the nervous system, which can result in severe impairment of physical and mental abilities. Unconsciousness can follow, and vomit may be inhaled, blocking the airway.

Common household poisons

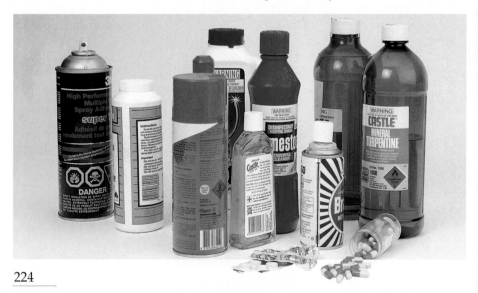

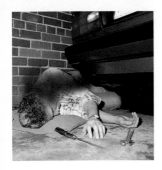

INHALED POISONS

Poisoning by inhalation occurs when a person breathes toxic fumes from a gas or substance. Such fumes usually cause breathing problems and can also result in headaches, nausea and dizziness, and affect the person's consciousness. Inhaled poisons include fumes from carbon monoxide (e.g. emitted by car engine or defective heating equipment), methane (e.g. in mines, wells, sewers), chlorine (e.g. in cleaners or swimming pool chemicals) and from paints, glues and industrial chemicals.

> **Warning**
>
> Anyone who is unconscious after inhaling poisonous gas or fumes needs oxygen with the greatest urgency.

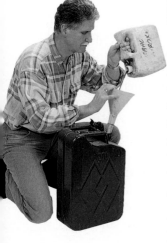

ABSORBED POISONS

Absorbed poisons enter the body through the skin or mucous membranes. These poisons include dry and wet chemicals, fertilisers, pesticides and any other substance that causes irritation and reddening of the skin at the point of contact. Contact with water makes some dry chemicals (e.g. dishwashing crystals) more toxic. These can be flushed away with running water.

INJECTED POISONS

Injected poisons enter the body as a result of a bite or sting from a spider, marine animal, fish, snake or insect. Drugs injected with a hypodermic needle or other sharp object cause many accidental and suicidal deaths each year.

MANAGEMENT OF POISONING

Signs and symptoms

The signs and symptoms of poisoning depend on the nature of the substance and, in some cases, how it entered the body. Any of the following may occur:

- abdominal pain
- drowsiness
- nausea and/or vomiting
- burning pain from mouth through to stomach
- difficulty breathing
- tight feeling in chest
- headache
- ringing in ears
- blurred vision
- smell of fumes
- odours on breath
- bite or injection marks, with or without local swelling
- contamination of skin
- change of skin colour; blueness around lips
- burns around and inside mouth or on tongue
- sudden collapse

Remember to:
- record the names of substances involved
- contact Poisons Information Service for specific advice on management
- send any containers and/or suicide notes with casualty to hospital
- send any vomit with casualty to hospital

MANAGEMENT OF POISONING—GENERAL

Unconscious casualty

1 Follow DRABC.

2 ☎ *Call 000 for an ambulance.*

3 ☎ *Call fire brigade* if atmosphere contaminated with smoke or gas.

Conscious casualty

1 Check for danger.

2 Listen to casualty; give reassurance but not advice.

3 Determine nature of substance, if possible, and record.

4 ☎ *Call 000 for an ambulance.*

5 ☎ *Call Poisons Information Centre—13 11 26.*

MANAGEMENT OF POISONING—SPECIFIC

Ingested poisons
For all ingested poisons, including a corrosive, petroleum-based, medicinal, or unknown substance:
- **DO NOT** induce vomiting
- **DO NOT** give anything by mouth
- wash corrosive substance off mouth and face with water, or wipe off

Inhaled poisons
- move casualty to fresh air
- loosen tight clothing

Absorbed poisons
- ask casualty to remove contaminated clothing
- shower skin clean
- launder contaminated clothes separately (be careful about your own skin contact)

Cyanide
- turn casualty on side
- if breathing stops, wash mouth and lips
- commence EAR (**DO NOT inhale casualty's expired air**)

Focus on Safety
PREVENTING POISONING

- handle and store all poisons with great care
- store out-of-reach of children
- only use childproof containers
- read instructions before use

Chemicals
- keep household products and medication in clearly labelled original containers
  - for identification
  - so directions for use are readily available
  - so precautions can be read
  - so instructions in case of poisoning are immediately available
- do not put harmful products in drink or food containers
- ventilate areas where toxic chemicals are used—open windows and doors
- wear protective clothing when using chemicals—gloves, face mask, eye protection, etc.
- do not use gas BBQs in a confined area
- if spraying chemicals outside
  - use lowest effective concentration
  - follow manufacturer's directions
  - spray when little or no wind

- make sure no-one is in area, especially children

Food
- do not use food which may be contaminated
- learn and use correct hygiene principles
- clean preparation areas and boards with bleach solution (1/2 tsp to 500 mls water)

Medication (medicine)
- read labels on medication carefully and take only as directed
- don't take someone else's medication
- do not leave medicines where children can get them
- do not take medication in front of children—they may imitate you
- take any unused or out-of-date medicines back to your chemist for disposal
- teach children to recognise warning labels and poison symbols

DO NOT dispose of unused poisonous substances by putting in garbage, emptying in sink, or flushing down toilet. DO return to chemist or supplier.

14

Bites and stings

Although most people fear snakes, snakebite is not a common occurrence in Australia and the amount of venom injected with a bite is not always dangerous. However, Australia's snakes are the most poisonous in the world, and the first aider is not able to assess how much venom has been injected. All snakebites must therefore be treated as life-threatening. Care has to be taken in the bush, in rural areas, and also in suburban areas close to grassland, bushland and rivers.

Animal bites and insect stings are painful and some are potentially lethal. More Australians die each year from bee stings than from shark attacks. Some marine animals, particularly those found in Australia's far north, are capable of deliveing a sting that is life-threatening.

This chapter discusses the first aid management techniques required for bites and stings.

BITES AND STINGS

Bites and stings occur frequently—in the garden, at the beach, at playgrounds, even in the home. Most bites and stings are relatively minor and, while painful, are not likely to result in the casualty's death. However, others can be deadly— bites from a poisonous snake (e.g. brown snake, tiger snake, or taipan), funnel-web spider and blue-ringed octopus, or stings from the cone shell and box jellyfish.

Venom injected directly into the bloodstream may work rapidly because it circulates quickly around the body. If injected just beneath the skin, the venom will act more slowly because it has to spread locally in the tissue fluids, then move into the lymphatic system before entering the blood- stream.

The venom of most Australian creatures moves in the body's tiny lymphatic vessels. The general effects are slow in onset, **as long as the casualty remains still.**

In treating snake and spider bites and insect stings, some important measures can be taken:
> ▶ **to slow movement of venom around body**— use a pressure immobilisation bandage
> ▶ **to manage pain**—use either icepacks/cold compresses, or hot fluids
> ▶ **to prevent further venom-release** into the body following stings by some marine animals (e.g. box jellyfish) **use vinegar**, which stops stinging-cells from firing and can be life-saving (though it has no effect on pain).

DRABC is the mainstay of management of all envenomations.

If the casualty has an allergic reaction to an otherwise non-lethal bite or sting, breathing and circulation could be affected and death may result if medical aid is not sought immediately. Be prepared to give EAR or CPR.

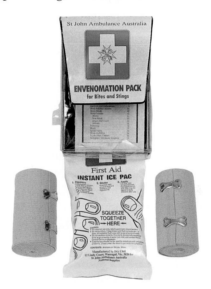

GENERAL PRINCIPLES FOR FIRST AID OF VENOMOUS BITES AND STINGS

1 Follow DRABC; avoid being bitten yourself.

DRABC

4 Seek medical aid (even if in doubt that the casualty has been bitten or stung).

2 Ask history of event, site of sting or bite, and where casualty was when bitten or stung.

5 Monitor breathing and circulation—be prepared to give CPR.

3 Carry out first aid quickly.

Pressure Immobilisation Bandaging

Pressure immobilisation is used for bites and stings from the following:
- snakes
- funnel-web spider
- mouse spider
- blue-ringed octopus
- box jellyfish
- cone shell

Note: For an allergic reaction to a bite or sting on a limb, apply a pressure immobilisation bandage.

A pressure immobilisation bandage applies pressure over wide areas of a limb. It compresses the tiny lymphatic vessels which carry most venoms. It is different from an arterial tourniquet which is applied only at one point and stops the pulse.

A pressure immobilisation bandage, together with splinting, is an effective form of management because the pressure over the bite area and limb slows the rate at which venom enters the circulation and is transported around the body. This delays the general effects of the venom.

DO NOT use pressure immobilisation for any of the following unless the casualty has a known allergy to the venom:
- red-back, white-tailed or recluse spider bite
- bee, wasp or ant stings
- tick bite
- bluebottle or Pacific man-of-war stings
- venomous fish stings (e.g. stonefish, stingray)

Pressure Immobilisation on a Limb

Use crepe or conforming roller bandage (about 10-15 cm wide); otherwise pantyhose or other material

- immediately apply a firm roller bandage starting just above the fingers or toes and moving upwards as far as can be reached up the limb
- apply firmly as for a sprained ankle

- immobilise the limb using a splint (use second bandage)
- check at fingers or toes for circulation
- keep the casualty and the limb at rest
- **DO NOT** remove splint or bandage once applied

Note: DO NOT allow the casualty to move.

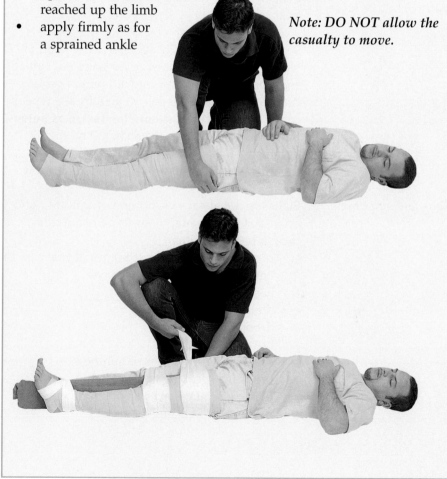

SNAKEBITE

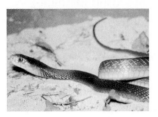

Taipan

Although some snakes (e.g. the carpet snake) are not venomous, Australia has the most lethal snakes in the world. The family of brown snakes has caused the greatest number of deaths in Australia, but a number of others, including the tiger snake, taipan and death adder, are very dangerous and their bite is always potentially fatal.

Snakes are not normally aggressive and tend to bite only when threatened or mishandled. Not all snakebites inject a significant amount of venom. As it is not always possible to identify the type of snake, **all snakebites should be treated as potentially lethal** and medical aid should be sought urgently. All major hospitals have a Venom Identification Kit to assist precise identification.

Signs and symptoms

Signs are not always visible and symptoms may only start to appear an hour or more after the person has been bitten.

- ▶ puncture marks or scratches (usually on a limb)
- ▶ nausea, vomiting and diarrhoea
- ▶ headache
- ▶ double or blurred vision
- ▶ drooping eyelids
- ▶ breathing difficulties
- ▶ drowsiness, giddiness or faintness
- ▶ problems speaking or swallowing
- ▶ pain or tightness in chest or abdomen
- ▶ respiratory weakness or arrest

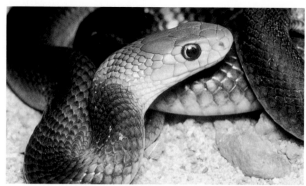

Common brown snake

Research has shown that the spread of snake venom depends on its absorption through the lymphatic system. Very little venom reaches the circulation, even after several hours, if a tight pressure immobilisation bandage and splint are applied, and if the casualty remains still. Venom affects different parts of the body but paralysis of the breathing muscles is the most serious effect and leads to death. If a child tells you that they have been bitten by a snake or spider, treat the incident seriously.

MANAGEMENT OF SNAKEBITE

1 Follow DRABC. **DRABC ▶**

2 Rest and calm the casualty.

3 Apply pressure immobilisation bandage.

4 Splint the bandaged limb.

5 **Ensure casualty does not move.**

6 ☎ *Call 000 for an ambulance.*

Warning

DO NOT wash venom off the skin as retained venom will assist identification.
DO NOT cut bitten area.
DO NOT try to suck venom out of wound.

DO NOT use a constrictive bandage (i.e. arterial tourniquet).
DO NOT try to catch the snake.

Spider Bites

Some spider bites are poisonous. Funnel-web spider venom has the potential to kill an adult. Red-back spiders inject venom which acts slowly and will not usually kill an adult. White-tailed spiders carry bacteria which may cause infection or skin ulceration.

Funnel-web spiders are black or dark brown and 2–3 cm in length. They rear back to bite and have large, strong fangs which can penetrate clothing and bite deeply if the skin is bare. A funnel-web hangs on and often has to be removed forcibly. Its bite can kill a child in minutes and an adult in a few hours if appropriate first aid and subsequent antivenene are not given.

Signs and symptoms

- sharp pain at bite site
- profuse sweating
- nausea, vomiting and abdominal pain

Additional symptoms of funnel-web spider bite:
- copious secretion of saliva
- confusion leading to coma
- muscular twitching and breathing difficulty

Additional symptoms of red-back spider bite:
- intense local pain which increases and spreads
- small hairs stand on end

Signs of white-tailed spider bite may include:
- burning sensation
- swelling
- blistering

MANAGEMENT OF SPIDER BITES

1 Follow DRABC. DRABC

2 Lie casualty down.

3 Calm casualty.

4 **Funnel-web/Mouse spider**
- apply pressure immobilisation bandage starting just above fingers or toes and as far up limb as possible
- ☎ *call 000 for an ambulance.*

Red-back
- apply cold pack/compress to area to lesson pain
- seek medical aid promptly.

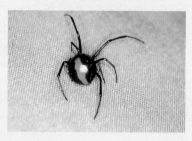
Red-back spider

White-tailed
- wash with soap and water
- apply cold pack/compress to relieve pain/discomfort
- seek medical aid if bite does not heal or skin ulceration occurs.

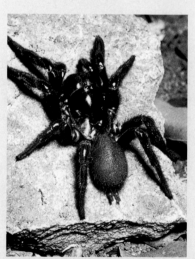
Funnel-web spider

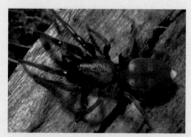
White-tailed spider

INSECT STINGS

While insect stings can be very painful, they are rarely fatal. They can, however, be dangerous for those who have an allergic reaction.

An allergic reaction can happen almost immediately and can result in blockage of the airway (anaphylactic shock) *(see p. 188 and p. 232).*

Signs and symptoms of allergic reaction to a sting

- rash, itching
- swollen eyelids, face, or neck tissues
- altered voice (e.g. high-pitched or 'crowing' sound)
- wheezing
- respiratory distress
- altered conscious state

Stings from **bees**, **wasps** and **ants** are always painful. Bee stings are usually left behind in the skin with the venom sac attached, and have to be removed (with a fingernail) with care. The European wasp can give multiple stings and inject a significant amount of venom.

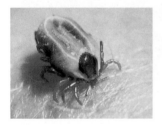

Ticks are very small. They attach themselves to the body and may be found in body crevices and hairy areas. The venom of the Australian paralysis tick—or scrub tick—can seriously affect people allergic to it. Ticks occur mainly along coastal eastern Australia from Queensland to northern Tasmania. The venom of other ticks may cause paralysis, especially in young children. Many ticks do not cause paralysis but may cause local irritation or a skin nodule.

Signs and symptoms
of insect stings

▶ pain at the site—sometimes extreme pain (European wasp)
▶ swelling and redness
▶ muscle weakness (tick)
▶ difficulty in breathing and swallowing (tick)

Note: Any of these symptoms can also be caused by an allergic reaction to any type of sting.

MANAGEMENT OF INSECT STINGS

1 Follow DRABC. **DRABC**

2 If severe allergic reaction:
☎ *call 000 for an ambulance.*

3 **Bee**
• remove sting—scrape sideways with your fingernail or the side of a sharp object (e.g. a knife).

Tick
• kill the tick with solvent-based insect repellent (pyrethrins).
• repeat after one minute
• after an hour check tick is dead—tick darkens and shrivels
• tick should brush off; if not, remove with tweezers
• try not to squeeze the tick while still attached.

4 Apply a cold compress to relieve pain if necessary.

5 Monitor ABC—give CPR if necessary.

Leech bite
• Leeches feed on the blood of humans and other vertebrates. Even when removed, the wound may take days to heal. The leech should not be pulled off as this may cause a severe wound. Instead, the leech may be removed by either the application of salt or touching it with a hot object e.g. an extinguished hot match. It can also be encouraged to let go by slicing it in half with a knife. Treat the wound as a normal bleeding injury.

MARINE BITES AND STINGS

Australia's tropical waters contain a number of animals whose stings can be life-threatening. Many beaches in Australia's north have large signs warning of the danger of stingers. No-one should swim on open mainland beaches in northern Australia during the 'stinger season' in summer (wet season).

The **box jellyfish** (found around the northern coast of Australia from Bundaberg on the east coast to Geraldton on the west) is extremely dangerous. The bites of the **blue-ringed octopus** (eastern Australia) and the **cone shell** (mostly tropical) can also be life-threatening.

Serious problems can also be caused by stings from the **Pacific man-of-war**, **Jimble jellyfish**, **Irukandji jellyfish**, **bullrout** (a fish found in inlets, rocky beaches, coral reefs and brackish

below left
Stonefish
below right
Box jellyfish

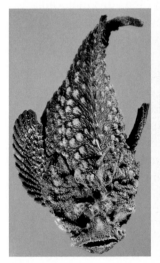

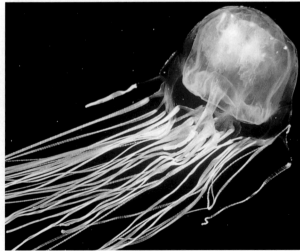

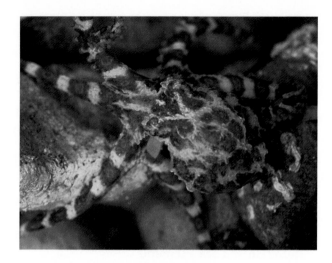

Blue-ringed octopus

estuaries), **cat fish**, **stonefish** (found on reefs and in estuaries) and **sea anemones**.

A sting to the chest or abdomen from a **stingray** is a serious medical emergency and requires immediate medical aid. (The stinging mechanism is attached half-way along the stingray's whip-like tail.) Signs and symptoms include immediate intense burning pain, bleeding from the wound and possibly breathing difficulty.

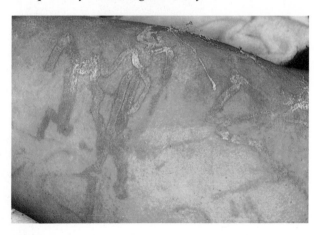

Sting from a box jellyfish

MANAGEMENT OF STINGING JELLYFISH
including Jimble and Irukandji jellyfish

1 Follow DRABC. In rescuing a casualty from the water, don't become enmeshed in tentacles yourself.

DRABC

2 Calm casualty; restrain casualty from rubbing stung area.

Bluebottle or Pacific man-of-war jellyfish and sea anemone

1 Gently pick off any adherent tentacles with tweezers or your fingers.

2 Apply cold packs or ice to reduce pain.

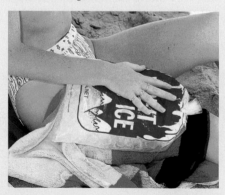

Box jellyfish

1 Flood the entire stung area with vinegar for at least 30 seconds.

2 Apply pressure immobilisation bandage but **NOT** over stings untreated with vinegar.

3 Splint the bandaged limb.

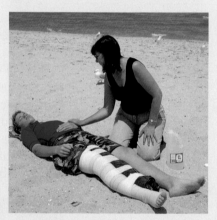

4 **Ensure casualty does not move.**

5 ☎ *Call 000 for an ambulance.*

Note: DO NOT wash the sting from bluebottle or Pacific man-of-war jellyfish with fresh water.

AT THE BEACH

Useful beach kit:

▶ 4 litres of vinegar (a necessity for those living in northern Australia)

▶ several broad elastic roller bandages

▶ small supply of ice or cold packs

▶ thermos of hot water

▶ way of communicating urgently (e.g. mobile phone)

☎ **For urgent advice concerning any marine envenomation you can call the Australian Venom Research Unit 24 hour advisory line – 03 9483 8204**

MANAGEMENT OF BLUE-RINGED OCTOPUS BITE AND CONE SHELL STING

1 Follow DRABC.

5 **Ensure casualty does not move.**

2 Calm casualty.

6 Give EAR if necessary.

3 Apply pressure immobilisation bandage.

7 ☎ **Call 000 for an ambulance.**

4 Splint the bandaged limb.

Note: The venom causes muscle paralysis leading to breathing failure and possibly death. EAR must be continued until medical aid is available, because, although long lasting, the paralysis will eventually abate.

MANAGEMENT OF FISH STINGS
including bullrout, catfish, stonefish, crown-of-thorns starfish, and stingray

1 Follow DRABC.

2 Calm casualty.

3 Remove any remaining sting barbs.

4 Place the casualty's stung foot or hand in hot water (as hot as the rescuer can comfortably tolerate).

5 ☎ *Call 000 for an ambulance.*

ANIMAL BITES

MANAGEMENT OF ANIMAL BITES

All animals (and humans) carry bacteria and other organisms in their mouths. Bites may puncture the skin. Untreated bites are highly likely to become infected.

1 Follow DRABC.

2 Control bleeding—use direct pressure and elevation.

3 Apply dressing, and bandage firmly.

4 Immobilise if bite on a limb.

5 Seek medical aid.

Bat bite

1 Handling of bats should be avoided.

2 Anyone either bitten or scratched by a bat should immediately:
- wash the wounds thoroughly with soap water
- promptly seek medical advice–regardless of the site or severity of the wound.

MANAGEMENT OF BITES AND STINGS REQUIRING URGENT MEDICAL ATTENTION

Box jellyfish	Cone shell, Blue-ringed octopus	Funnel-web spider/Mouse spider	Red-back spider	Snake
DRABC	DRABC	DRABC	DRABC	DRABC
☎ *Call 000*	☎ *Call 000*	☎ *Call 000*		☎ *Call 000*
			Apply ice-pack	
	EAR as breathing difficulty progresses		Seek medical aid	
Douse area with vinegar for 30+ secs	and continue until paralysis abates			
Pressure immobilisation (above stung area only, if no vinegar)	Pressure immobilisation	Pressure immobilisation		Pressure immobilisation
Immobilise limb—splint	Immobilise limb—splint	Immobilise limb—splint		Immobilise limb—splint

NOTE: All allergic reactions require urgent medical attention. If casualty has medication for allergy, ensure it is taken at once.

MANAGEMENT OF OTHER BITES AND STINGS

Jellyfish— Bluebottle, Jimble, Pacific man-of-war, Irukandji, sea anemones	Centipede, Scorpion, Ant	Fish stings, Crown-of-thorns starfish	Tick	Bee	Wasp/ hornet, European wasp
Pick off tentacles		DRABC Extract barb if possible	Kill tick Remove with tweezers	Remove sting	
Apply cold pack	Apply cold pack			Apply cold pack	Apply cold pack
		Apply hot fluid			
DO NOT wash with fresh water		☎ *Call 000*			

NOTE: All allergic reactions require urgent medical attention. If a casualty has medication for allergy, ensure it is taken at once.

FOCUS ON SAFETY
PREVENTING BITES AND STINGS

Preventing insect and spider bites
- avoid using or wearing products that attract insects
- cover exposed areas of the body
- wear an insect repellent when outdoors
- arrange for safe removal of any nest of stinging insects near your home
- do not panic if a bee or wasp comes near you—teach your children not to panic
- wear gloves when gardening
- teach your children to avoid touching spiders

Preventing tick bites
- wear a long-sleeved shirt with a firm collar and cuffs and tuck pants into socks or boots when walking through the bush or long grass
- check your body for ticks after walking in the bush

Preventing snakebite
- make a lot of noise when walking in the bush
- always wear shoes outside
- be aware of snakes' habits
- don't put hands or feet where you can't see what is there
- don't put your hand into a hollow log
- don't reach into long grass
- don't pick up a 'stick' unless you have checked it carefully
- if climbing, don't reach up and put your hand on a ledge of rock without looking first
- teach children to keep clear of snakes
- keep grass cut around house
- be extremely wary of all snakes—keep away!

Preventing animal bites
- teach children how to respond to and approach dogs
- when camping, store food and drink out-of-reach of animals
- do not feed wild animals

Preventing marine animal bites and stings
- do not step on bluebottles washed up on the sand
- do not swim in waters where there are warning signs
- do not touch marine creatures in the water
- do not swim in creeks and rivers known to be crocodile habitat
- wear sandshoes and wetsuit or bodystocking when necessary

15

Lifting and moving casualties

CONTENTS

Moving a casualty from an accident scene poses dangers for the first aider as well as for the casualty. Whenever possible, apply first aid without moving casualty from the scene.

However, there may be dangers such as fire or explosion, or it may not be possible to give first aid due to the casualty's position. It may also be necessary to transport the casualty to a medical facility.

If it is necessary to move a casualty, use a method that poses the least amount of risk—both to yourself and the casualty. This chapter outlines the ways in which a casualty can be moved with maximum safety.

LIFTING AND MOVING CASUALTIES

A first aider should always try to give first aid where the casualty is found, as moving can result in further injury or make existing injuries worse. **A casualty should only be moved if there is immediate danger**—such as from a collapsing structure, traffic hazards, fire or poisonous fumes.

MOVING A CASUALTY

When it is necessary to move a casualty, do so by the quickest means available; then, while waiting for medical aid to arrive, make sure:
- there is no further danger
- the casualty has a clear airway and is able to breathe
- bleeding is controlled

If injuries are serious, it is best to transport the casualty to hospital by ambulance as improvised transport may reduce the chances of survival. However, an ambulance may not be available.

Before moving the casualty consider
- whether you can handle size and weight of the person without injury to either of you
- what other help is available
- type and seriousness of injuries
- terrain to be crossed
- distance casualty has to be moved
- whether a neck stabilising collar should be applied before movement
- if travel or motion sickness may make casualty worse

LIFTING A CASUALTY

If you need to lift a casualty, try to ensure as much comfort as possible so neither you nor the casualty sustain injury or strain.

When lifting, remember to

▶ bend at the knees
▶ keep your back straight and head up
▶ keep in a balanced position
▶ keep your centre of gravity low
▶ hold the weight close to your body for stability
▶ take small steps
▶ work as a team—someone must take role of leader

LIFTING A CASUALTY—GENERAL MANAGEMENT

Conscious casualty

1 Follow DRABC.

2 Manage all injuries and immobilise fractures.

3 Tell casualty what you are intending to do.

4 Seek casualty's help and cooperation.

5 Make sure casualty feels secure.

6 Always use help to lift if available.

7 Hold casualty firmly.

8 Avoid risks where possible.

EMERGENCY MOVES AND LIFTS

A move is successful if it is carried out without injuring yourself or without causing further injury to the casualty. Different methods are used to move the casualty depending on the circumstances and whether there is anyone to help.

A casualty who is conscious and not seriously injured may be able to walk away from the danger with your help. However, **a casualty who is unconscious or seriously injured** will need to be moved from danger using one of the following methods:

Ankle drag

▶ used for people too large or heavy to carry or move in any other way

▶ preferably used for dragging over smooth ground

▶ less risk of back injury to first aider

▶ maintains traction on the body to keep bone ends apart if the casualty has a fracture

▶ **DO NOT use** for lower leg injuries

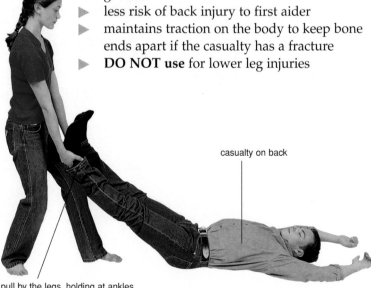

casualty on back

pull by the legs, holding at ankles

Arm drag

- used as an alternative to the ankle drag
- used for casualty with a suspected head or neck injury, if they **must** be moved from danger
- can result in back injury for first aider

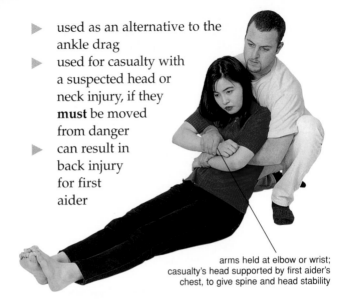

arms held at elbow or wrist; casualty's head supported by first aider's chest, to give spine and head stability

Clothes drag

- used for someone suspected of having a head, spine or other major injury
- head is cradled by clothing and first aider's hands
- exhausting and can result in back strain for first aider

arms kept on ground, head supported by first aider's forearms—to prevent aggravation to neck injury

open top buttons of shirt or jacket

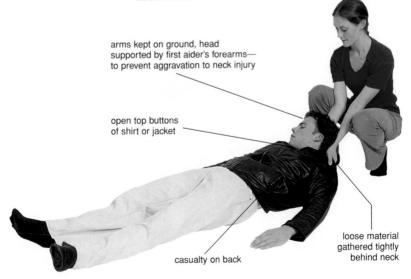

loose material gathered tightly behind neck

casualty on back

251

MOVING A CASUALTY WITH NO ASSISTANCE

The cradle

The cradle is used to carry a child or light casualty. (If the casualty is heavier than anticipated, seek assistance.) When lifting the casualty:

1 Ensure your back is kept straight.

2 Use your leg muscles to rise.

3 Arch backwards slightly to counterbalance weight.

Small children when unconscious are best carried with one arm under knees and other arm around and supporting neck—this gives control of head and allows it to be lowered for drainage of vomit, saliva etc. Depending on child's size, first aider uses either hand to steady child's crossed arms on chest or abdomen.

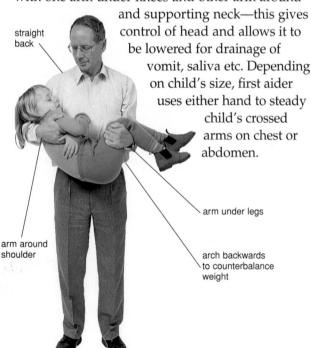

straight back

arm around shoulder

arm under legs

arch backwards to counterbalance weight

The human crutch

The human crutch is used when a casualty has an injured leg or foot but is able to walk on the uninjured leg with your assistance (casualty may also be able to take some weight on injured leg).

1 Help casualty stand.

2 Place yourself on injured side.

3 Take weight of casualty's injured side on your shoulders.

4 Step off together, leading with your inside foot.

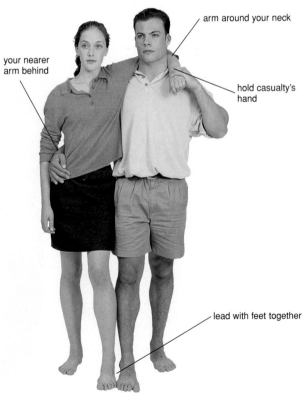

your nearer arm behind

arm around your neck

hold casualty's hand

lead with feet together

253

Piggy-back

Piggy-back is used for conscious patients with lower limb injuries who are able to hold on with their arms.

1 Help casualty stand.

2 Crouch down in front of casualty with your back to them.

3 Straighten up only when casualty is in position.

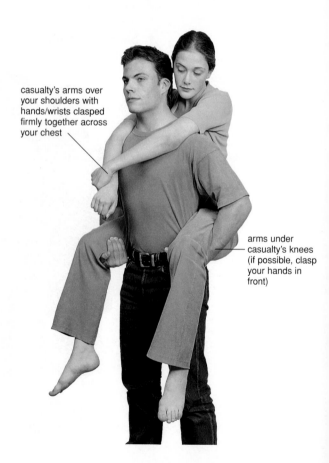

casualty's arms over your shoulders with hands/wrists clasped firmly together across your chest

arms under casualty's knees (if possible, clasp your hands in front)

Lift and drag

The lift and drag is used to drag a heavy, helpless casualty from danger.

1 Tie casualty's wrists together.

2 With casualty on back, kneel astride them.

3 Place your head and one arm through casualty's arms.

4 Crawl on hands and knees, lifting casualty's head and shoulders clear of ground.

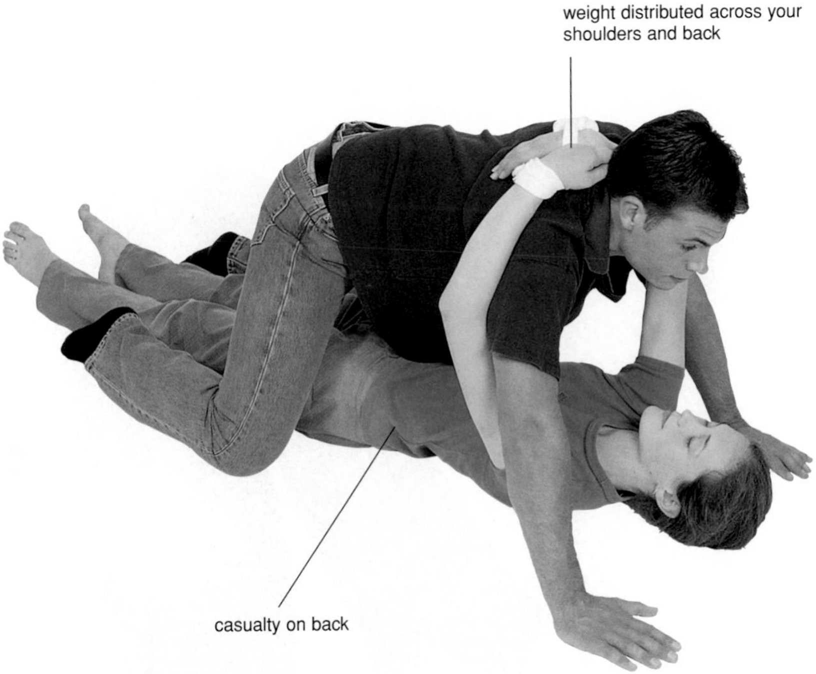

weight distributed across your shoulders and back

casualty on back

Warning

Never take the casualty's weight solely on your neck.

Fireman's lift and carry   Fireman's lift and carry is used for casualties who are unconscious or helpless and are not too heavy for the first aider.

1 Lie casualty on back in front of you.

2 Pull casualty up by wrists and over your shoulder.

3 Adjust casualty's weight for balance over shoulder.

4 Pass hand between casualty's legs; grasp casualty's wrist.

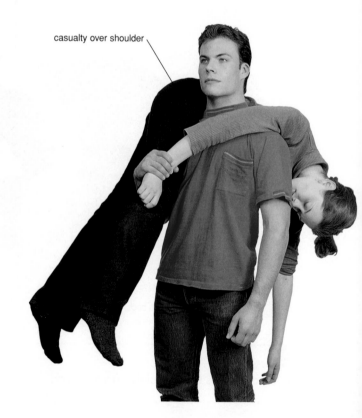

casualty over shoulder

MOVING A CASUALTY WITH ASSISTANCE

Two-person human crutch

The two-person human crutch is used for a casualty who can support weight on one leg without making the injury worse (may also be able to take some weight on other leg).

1 Help casualty stand.

2 Stand one each side of casualty.

3 First aiders take casualty's arms around their shoulders and hold wrists.

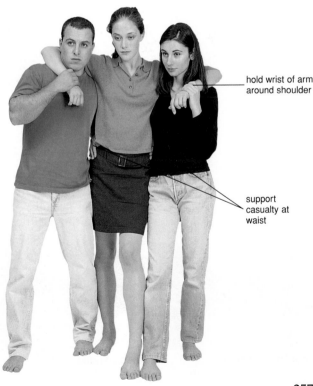

hold wrist of arm around shoulder

support casualty at waist

**Four-handed,
three-handed and
two-handed seats**

▷ **four-handed seat**—used when casualty is able
to use one or both arms to help

▷ **three-handed seat**—used when one leg needs
supporting

▷ **two-handed seat**—used for any conscious
casualty who can be carried in a sitting position,
but needs support from both first aiders

For each hand seat, both first aiders will need to:

1 Hold each other's wrists firmly (left to right;
right to left).

2 Squat down to allow casualty to sit on hands.

3 Rise together to lift casualty.

4 Step off on inside foot together.

5 Use crossover step to walk.

Remember:

▷ the higher casualty is lifted the easier carrying
will be

▷ do not have your arms straight when placed
under the casualty's thighs as this makes
carrying more difficult

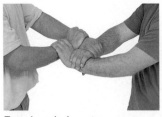
Four-handed seat

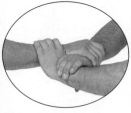
Three-handed seat

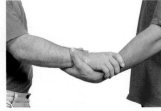
Two-handed seat

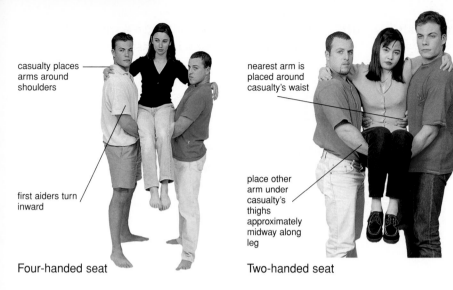

casualty places arms around shoulders

first aiders turn inward

Four-handed seat

nearest arm is placed around casualty's waist

place other arm under casualty's thighs approximately midway along leg

Two-handed seat

Fore and aft lift

The fore and aft lift may have to be used when operating in a narrow area where there is not room to use a hand seat.

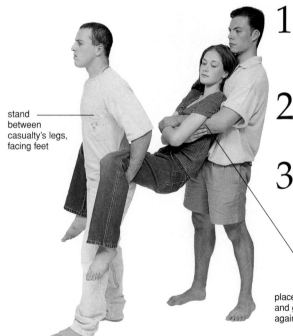

stand between casualty's legs, facing feet

place arms under armpits and grasp casualty's wrists against their chest

1 Both first aiders bend at the knees, backs as straight as possible, and take hold of the casualty.

2 Casualty's head and shoulders are raised before grasping from behind.

3 First aiders rise together and walk in step.

259

Fore and aft chair lift

The fore and aft chair lift is used when a chair is available, with a conscious casualty who has a serious injury.

1   First aiders place casualty in chair.

2   Kneel down to grasp legs/back of chair (front first aider facing away from casualty).

3   First aiders rise together and walk in step.

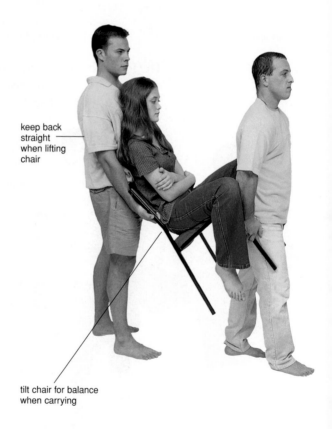

keep back straight when lifting chair

tilt chair for balance when carrying

STRETCHERS

Using a stretcher is the safest way to move those who are seriously injured as the chance of further injury is reduced.

Note: If moving the casualty means any possibility of adverse effects, do not move. Wait until an ambulance arrives.

It is important to:
- test stretcher for strength and security
- keep stretcher as level as possible
- keep movement to necessary minimum
- correctly position casualty on stretcher (depending on injuries and condition)
- fasten casualty securely to stretcher
- protect casualty from weather when necessary

If the casualty has a head injury, is unconscious, or is likely to vomit, place in recovery position on stretcher. Work as quickly and carefully as possible, to ensure safety.

If the casualty has a suspected spinal injury or is unconscious:
- avoid putting pressure on localised areas
- use padding (e.g. sandbags, clothing or blankets) to keep head in a stable position
- **DO NOT** allow the neck or spine to move or be twisted; use cervical collar or improvise
- remove coins, keys etc. from casualty's pockets

Securing casualty to a stretcher

When securing casualty to a stretcher, make sure the bandages do not aggravate injuries.

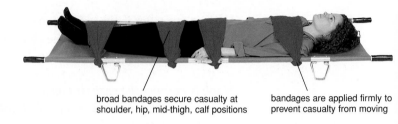

broad bandages secure casualty at shoulder, hip, mid-thigh, calf positions

bandages are applied firmly to prevent casualty from moving

Blanketing a stretcher

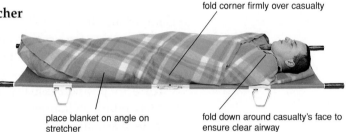

fold corner firmly over casualty

place blanket on angle on stretcher

fold down around casualty's face to ensure clear airway

Loading stretcher without using blankets

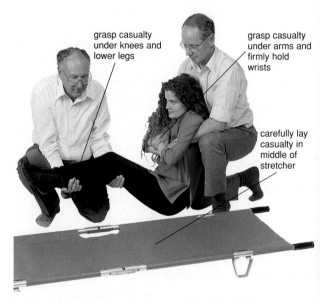

grasp casualty under knees and lower legs

grasp casualty under arms and firmly hold wrists

carefully lay casualty in middle of stretcher

Note: For loading stretcher using blanket, see pages 266–7.

Loading and lifting stretcher using available bystanders as assistants

When possible use bystanders to assist with the lift. This shares the load, reduces risk of damage to any lifter and avoids twisting with heavy loads. It is also much more comfortable for the casualty.

The first aider should organise and take charge of the lift. The first aider should also be responsible for an unconscious casualty's head and airway or for the injured part if the casualty is conscious.

If four people share the lift of a 60 kg casualty (an average weight for a woman), each will only lift 15 kg. The actual lift should be directed by the first aider, giving the instruction that on the command 'lift', all will lift.

THE JORDON FRAME

The Jordon frame is used for casualties with suspected spinal or other major injuries, if the casualty is in a position where the frame can be placed around them. Because the stretcher has a rigid frame, it can be used to lift an injured person with little or no disturbance to the injuries. (It is not used for transporting the casualty.)

Assembling the Jordon frame

1 Place frame around casualty—top lug in line with casualty's ear.

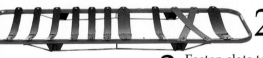

2 Slide plastic slats underneath casualty—tapered end first.

3 Fasten slats to frame.

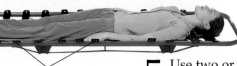

4 Adjust position and tension of each slat as necessary.

placement of slats on Jordon frame with casualty on it

5 Use two or more first aiders to lift casualty.

THE SCOOP STRETCHER

The scoop stretcher enfolds and closes shut underneath a casualty in the position in which they were found. The stretcher:

▶ minimises possibility of complicating injuries
▶ is adjustable to casualty's physique
▶ can be manoeuvred through a narrow space
▶ can be lifted and carried by two or more first aiders

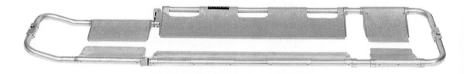

In difficult manoeuvring positions, the casualty should be strapped to the stretcher, a special velcro strap being used to immobilise the head and neck. Take care to:

▶ avoid pressure on localised areas
▶ use padding
▶ remove coins, keys etc. from casualty's pockets
▶ use sandbags or similar padding to maintain head in a stable position (use cervical collar if available)
▶ lift stretcher from sides if casualty is heavy
▶ ensure casualty is on back and the head supported by a thin pillow so that you can monitor the airway closely

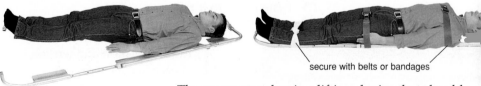

secure with belts or bandages

The scoop stretcher is a lifting device that should be removed when the casualty is placed on a standard stretcher, trolley or bed.

IMPROVISED STRETCHERS

It is possible to prepare an improvised stretcher using a ladder, door, table, plank, or poles, together with coats, sacks, blankets, or bandages.

When using a coat, turn the sleeves inside out, pass the poles through them and pin the coat ends around the poles. A cross piece, lashed to each pole at the head and foot, will make the stretcher more comfortable and effective.

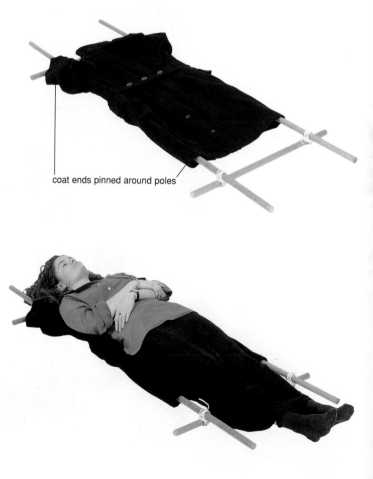

coat ends pinned around poles

THE BLANKET LIFT

A simple blanket can make an excellent lifting device. However, this lift is not used for those whom you suspect have a neck or spinal injury.

1 Place blanket on ground.

2 Roll blanket lengthwise for half its width.

3 Roll casualty onto uninjured side.

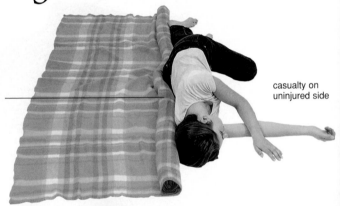

place rolled section of blanket up against casualty's back

casualty on uninjured side

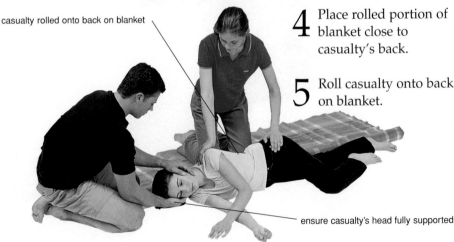

casualty rolled onto back on blanket

4 Place rolled portion of blanket close to casualty's back.

5 Roll casualty onto back on blanket.

ensure casualty's head fully supported

6 Unroll the blanket.

Loading stretcher using blanket

7 To lift:
- roll up edges of blanket until alongside casualty (edges act as handles for lifters)
- grasp rolled edges firmly
- all lifters rise at same time.

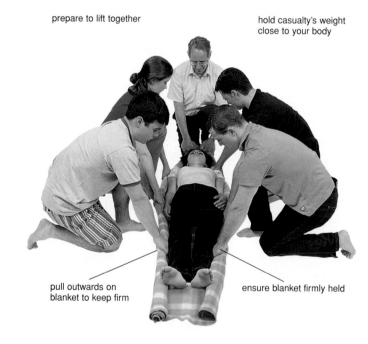

prepare to lift together

hold casualty's weight close to your body

pull outwards on blanket to keep firm

ensure blanket firmly held

8 One lifter takes control.

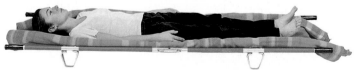

Casualty lifted and placed on stretcher

Transporting a Casualty to Medical Aid

You may have to drive a casualty to medical aid.
If so, remember:

▶ casualty still needs the same care as if they were not being moved

▶ the nature of casualty's injuries will determine appropriate vehicle to use (if you have a choice)

▶ do not exceed speed limit

▶ if necessary travel slowly to ensure that casualty's injuries are not made worse

▶ the most experienced first aider stays with casualty to monitor airway

Casualties suffering from the following conditions must always be transported on a stretcher:

▶ head injuries

▶ spinal injuries

▶ abdominal injuries

▶ lower limb injuries

▶ embedded foreign bodies or penetrating wounds to the eye

Casualties with minor injuries and some upper limb injuries may be moved (preferably only short distances) sitting in a car, provided the injured parts are adequately supported.

Road traffic accidents and triage

16

In Australia more people die in road accidents than in any other type of accident. Road transport injury is the most common form of accidental death in the middle years of life.

Over a lifetime, everyone will witness or be involved in a traffic accident; one in every twenty people will be involved in a major accident. Anyone could be required to give first aid to those injured. This chapter outlines how to deal with such a situation.

In a road accident—or other major accident or natural disaster—in which there is more than one casualty, a system known as triage is used to classify casualties and set priorities for first aid management and evacuation. The aim is for the most good to be done for the maximum number of people. Basic principles of triage are outlined in this chapter.

ROAD TRAFFIC ACCIDENTS

At a major traffic accident, a first aider should know how to manage the situation. In urban areas, emergency services usually arrive quickly, but in remote rural locations a first aider may have to cope without assistance for an extended time.

Safety is the first consideration—safety of the casualty, the first aider and bystanders. Casualties may be on or off the road or in a vehicle. They can be in danger unless the site is made safe. This involves:

▶ assessing danger
▶ taking control of accident site
▶ protecting casualty, first aiders and other personnel (e.g. by warning oncoming traffic)

ASSESSING THE DANGER

At an accident site, first aiders must make an assessment of the possible danger to themselves and to any casualties.

Dangers to look for include:

▶ other traffic
▶ fire or fumes
▶ damaged vehicles
▶ spilt fuel or chemicals
▶ fallen or damaged overhead powerlines
▶ high-voltage electricity
▶ distraught or potentially violent people
▶ unstable structures (e.g. powerlines or buildings)

Other traffic

Other traffic is always of primary concern. The accident site has to be protected so that no further accidents occur. To warn other vehicles:

1 Safely park a car at a suitable distance from accident.

2 Put on hazard lights.

3 If at night, use headlights to illuminate scene.

4 Ask bystanders to warn and control oncoming vehicles.

Fire

Fire can start in any badly damaged vehicle, particularly if electrical wiring is damaged or fuel spilt. To prevent fires:

1 Switch off vehicle's ignition.

2 Shut off emergency fuel switch of a diesel vehicle.

3 Prevent anyone smoking near accident site.

Obtain a fire extinguisher if possible, and have it ready. If there is a fire under the bonnet of a vehicle, release the bonnet catch (if possible), but do not open the bonnet fully. Aim the fire extinguisher through the gap towards the flames.

Fumes

Fumes from leaking petrol can cause an explosion. Bystanders should be kept well away and no naked flames or smoking allowed.

Damaged vehicle

A damaged vehicle can be dangerous so take precautions including:

1 Put on handbrake.

2 Put vehicle in gear (if not already).

3 Place blocks against wheels.

Spilt fuel or chemicals

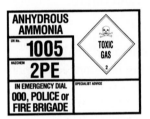

Where an accident involves a vehicle carrying hazardous materials, the rule is to stay clear of the accident scene. However, emergency services must be notified and care taken by the first aider to secure the safety of the scene. Without putting yourself in danger, note:

▶ clouds of vapour
▶ spilt liquids, bottles, gas cylinders
▶ unusual odours

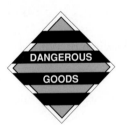

Vehicles containing hazardous substances will have display notices or signs indicating the contents. When notifying emergency services, give:

▶ code number (HAZCHEM Emergency Action Code)
▶ type of sign

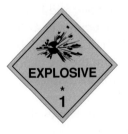

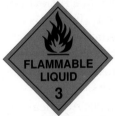

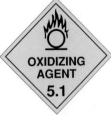

Avoid contact with these substances and stay upwind to avoid breathing in any toxic fumes.

High-voltage electricity, fallen powerlines

High-voltage electricity can be a serious hazard at an accident site. If a car has hit a light or electricity pole, high-voltage powerlines can be knocked down and may even come into contact with the vehicle. If this has happened:

▶ remain at least 6 metres from any cable (high-voltage electricity can arc up to 6 metres)

▶ ensure bystanders do not go within 6 metres of cable

▶ call emergency services

▶ **DO NOT** attempt to move cable

▶ **DO NOT** go near a vehicle or try to remove a person from a vehicle being touched by a high-voltage cable

There is considerable risk that a vehicle with a fallen cable touching it could catch fire. If it becomes necessary, due to fire—or other external life-threatening situation—for anyone in the vehicle to get out, they should do so **only if they can jump clear without touching the vehicle and the ground at the same time**. Otherwise, they will act as an earth for the electricity and may be killed.

In most situations, anyone inside the vehicle should be told to remain there until the danger from the electrical cable has been removed.

Distraught or potentially violent person

The distraught or potentially violent person may be experiencing a significant emotional reaction to the accident, or a loved-one may be seriously injured, trapped in the vehicle, or even dead. These people need special consideration at a major accident scene. They have to be cared for, and perhaps prevented from interfering with the management and removal of other casualties. If people at the accident scene are physically uninjured, but very agitated, or preventing the first aider from attending to serious injuries, they need to be removed gently but firmly. A suitable bystander can be recruited to escort them, then stay to try to calm and reassure them.

CONTROL OF THE ACCIDENT SITE

Control of an accident site aims to ensure:

▶ casualty is protected from further injury
▶ first aider and caregivers are protected from injury
▶ easier access for emergency services
▶ more efficient treatment and evacuation to hospital
▶ easier assessment of priorities for casualty management (triage)

If the site is well controlled, more lives can be saved.

Resources available at an accident site

Bystanders can be an asset. They can:

▶ call emergency services
▶ warn traffic to slow down or stop
▶ run messages for people giving aid
▶ care for physically uninjured casualties
▶ help give CPR
▶ help with triage
▶ secure area from onlookers
▶ clear road to allow access by emergency vehicles
▶ help lift casualties

Other cars can be used to warn oncoming vehicles there is an accident ahead. Cars not involved in the accident or not being used to warn oncoming traffic should be cleared from the site if possible. **Phones, two-way radios** and **CB radios** are often available in cars, taxis, interstate transports, and courier vehicles. These can be used to contact emergency services.

NOTIFICATION OF ACCIDENT

Any traffic accident should be reported to the emergency services as soon as possible. Call 000 for an ambulance and police and any other service required. If there is a damaged powerline tell the telephone operator, to ensure that the electricity authority is also contacted.

EMERGENCY NUMBER PRIORITY—*CALL 000*

What emergency service do you need?
> Always ask for an ambulance first, then police.

Who else is needed at accident site?
> *Is there a danger from high voltage wires?*
>> Ask for electricity authority to be contacted.
>
> *Is there a danger from spilled chemicals?*
>> Ask for fire brigade.
>
> *Is there a danger from fire?*
>> Ask for fire brigade.

It is important to be able to give emergency services all the information they require about the location of the accident, number of casualties and types of injuries etc.

In a city or town, give:	In a rural area, give:	If a road accident, give:

• street number
• street
• landmarks
  (e.g. cross street)
• suburb
• city/town
	• distance from
	  intersection/landmark/
	  roadside number
	• road
	• area
	• nearest city/town
	• landmark
		• number of people
		  involved
		• is anybody trapped?
		• are powerlines
		  involved?
		• other hazards

MANAGEMENT OF ACCIDENT SITE

An accident scene can quickly fall into confusion if no-one takes time to organise. Time can be lost in getting treatment and lives may even be lost. An accident scene is best handled if someone takes responsibility for management. As a trained first aider, it may be more effective for you to manage the entire situation than to help only one person.

TYPES OF INJURIES

The injuries you are likely to have to deal with will vary according to the type of accident. Airway blockage is the most common problem with those involved in an accident, as casualties are thrown forward by the force of the impact. The most common serious injuries are to the head and chest for adults and to the head for children.

Pedestrians often have multiple injuries. Head and spinal injuries are common and often fatal. If run over, the pedestrian may have a crushed chest, abdomen or pelvis. There may also be injuries from being dragged under a car.

Bicyclists have a high risk of head injury, especially if not wearing a helmet. They often have severe arm and leg injuries and sustain similar injuries to pedestrians when hit by a vehicle.

Motorcyclists are the most likely of all road users to suffer a spinal injury resulting in paralysis. They may also have large areas of skin stripped off by the road or other hard surface. These injuries are particularly prone to infection because they contain a lot of embedded dirt and debris.

REMOVAL OF HELMETS

A traffic accident may involve someone who is wearing a motorcycle helmet or other type of protective headgear. The helmet should be removed **only if absolutely necessary**—e.g. if the casualty needs resuscitation. Casualties should remove their own helmets whenever possible. However it may be necessary for a helmet to be removed in order to deal with injuries.

MANAGEMENT OF HELMET REMOVAL

Note: Removal of helmets should be performed by two people.

1 Place the casualty on back, supporting the head (avoid moving head up, down or to the side).

2 Unfasten the chin strap—cut if necessary.

Open face helmets

3 Pull sides of helmet apart to take pressure away from casualty's head—have someone support casualty's neck if possible.

4 Gently lift helmet back and up off head.

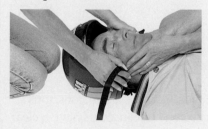

Full face helmets

3 Gently insert your fingers under rim, while supporting the neck and holding jaw firmly.

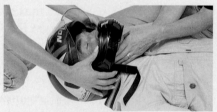

4 A second first aider should tilt helmet backwards, lifting front to clear chin.

5 Tilt helmet forward to clear base of skull and lift helmet off.

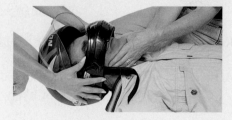

PRIORITIES AT ACCIDENT SITE

In dealing with the casualties of an accident, the DRABC Action Plan remains the first priority. However, an accident brings in other factors that have to be considered. The following guidelines will help:

Hazards

▶ make sure everyone at accident site is protected, by safely parking your car and putting hazard lights on

▶ light up a night accident scene with headlights

▶ assess scene for other dangers and remove if possible

▶ move casualty from danger if this is more appropriate (e.g. if there is a fire)

Assessment

▶ make a rapid assessment of:
  - how many casualties
  - severity of injuries
  - any dangerous circumstances to report
  - whether anyone is trapped

▶ ensure all occupants of cars are accounted for

Help

▶ ☎ *call 000 for an ambulance and police*
  - consider need to call other services (e.g. fire brigade, electricity authority)

Follow the remainder of DRABC Action Plan to manage casualties:

Response

- are casualties conscious or unconscious?

Airway

- ensure all casualties who are unconscious or likely to become unconscious have a clear airway. Remember no other injury takes precedence over a clear airway!

Breathing • ensure all casualties are breathing; manage casualty who has difficulty breathing

Circulation • ensure all casualties have a pulse; manage casualty who has no pulse

Bleeding • manage casualties who are bleeding

TRIAGE

Triage is the classification and sorting of casualties for the purpose of management and evacuation, according to the degree of urgency. The aim is for the most good to be done for the largest number of people. It only applies to a situation where there is more than one casualty.

SMALL ACCIDENTS (2–3 CASUALTIES)

The first aider will have to assess each casualty's injuries and situation (e.g. whether trapped in a vehicle) to determine an order of priority for first aid management.

Your decisions about which vehicle is most likely to contain casualties with serious injuries, and about which of the injured are most likely to need urgent attention, may literally be a matter of life or death. Such decisions frequently need to be made on the basis of limited information and in situations of critical urgency.

Main principles

To decide the urgency of each casualty's need for care and evacuation, the first aider needs to be able to assess injuries according to a plan. In making such decisions, two main principles apply:

▶ **acute needs override long-term outcomes**—a casualty with a fractured spine will generally have lower priority for evacuation than a casualty with internal abdominal bleeding
▶ **life takes precedence over limb**—a casualty who is not breathing has priority over a casualty who is bleeding

Remember: Airway management has highest priority.

MAJOR TRAFFIC ACCIDENTS

A major traffic accident may involve multiple vehicles, a coach or bus, etc.

At any accident site, first aid management will be limited by the resources available. This is particularly the case when there is a large number of casualties or when there will be a significant time before emergency services arrive. In rural areas, people involved in a traffic accident are at greater risk; hence the importance of calling emergency services as soon as possible.

Multiple vehicle accidents tend to occur in daylight and where traffic flow is dense. A major traffic accident will usually involve a number of casualties. The site can become congested with trained first aiders, onlookers, and emergency services personnel. If you are able to establish a site control centre and to plan management, you will make the work of the emergency services easier and enable a more efficient handover of control.

Site control centre

A site control centre should be:
- ▶ as near accident site as possible
- ▶ elevated so you can see whole accident site
- ▶ easily reached

Triage areas should be distinctly marked and the site control centre well protected. It should be positioned so as to provide good access both to casualties and evacuation routes.

Ranking casualties

Expert specialist triage (by salaried ambulance services) at a major accident site involves ranking casualties by attaching labels. For the first aider, the process is less formalised but the concept remains the same. It is important to remember that a casualty is always in a changing, not static, condition. This is especially important with head and abdominal injuries in which deterioration can occur.

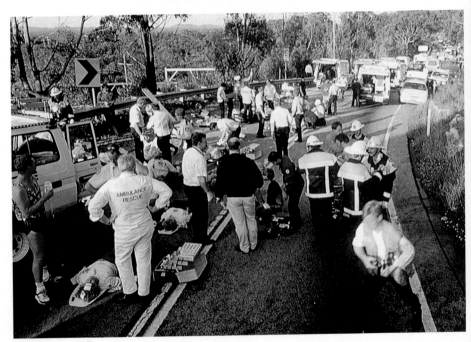

When there is a number of casualties, they are grouped into four main categories for evacuation from the accident site:

Group 1

Casualties with minor injuries—would not normally need medical treatment (e.g. minor bruises or abrasions, fright, slight headache).

These casualties should be registered, then instructed to leave the accident area unassisted or with a friend, to seek medical aid or return home.

Group 2

Casualties requiring medical treatment but not immediate hospitalisation—(e.g. ankle sprains, large bruises and abrasions, back strain).

These casualties can be evacuated to their homes after registration and instructed to seek early treatment from their own medical practitioner.

Note: Casualties classified in the preceding two groups ought, if possible, receive appropriate first aid management prior to evacuation. However, they should not be allowed to crowd an accident site or delay attention to the more urgent cases. They are more likely to receive early medical treatment at home or at a private doctor's surgery than they are if transported to the hospital receiving the more seriously injured.

Group 3

Casualties who require early transport to hospital—some will need urgent surgery to survive whereas others can wait.

This group can be further subdivided into priority cases:

Priority 1—Requiring urgent transport to hospital

- breathing difficulties (e.g. flail chest, collapsed lung/lungs, obstructed airway)
- severe bleeding, abdominal injury with signs of shock, open fractures, crush injuries, burns to 30% or more of body surface
- head injuries and deteriorating level of consciousness
- multiple injuries

Priority 2—May require surgery within a few hours

- unconscious with a clear airway
- abdominal injury without signs of shock
- large wounds where bleeding has been controlled
- burns to 10–30% of body surface
- fractures or dislocation of major joints

Priority 3—Most will require surgery when practicable

- closed fractures
- facial injuries without airway obstruction
- eye injury
- minor wounds
- burns to less than 10% of body surface
- spinal injury

Group 4

Casualties clinically dead and those who will probably die before reaching hospital—e.g. those who have been decapitated, have massive head or torso injuries, have been cut in half, whose brain and skull have been very severely damaged or who have been incinerated.

These casualties are the last to be evacuated. They should be managed with dignity and protection.

The triage officer must not jeopardise the survival of those with a possibility of recovery by using ambulance and hospital resources for the untreatable, because of fear of making an error.

OTHER TYPES OF ACCIDENTS

The principles of triage apply to other types of accidents involving a number of casualties—explosion, collapse of a building or scaffolding or some other industrial mishap. In such an incident, the first aider may have to manage a team effort to give first aid to the casualties.

Because of the danger of further casualties from secondary explosion and building collapse, and the need to minimise congestion, it is important to remove casualties from the accident site as soon as possible.

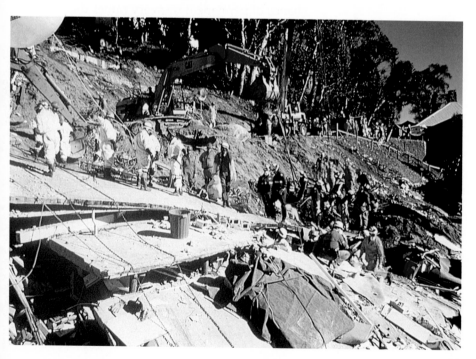

NATURAL DISASTERS

In most cases where there is a large number of casualties, ambulance and hospital services are able to cope. In certain situations however (e.g. an earthquake, cyclone or major explosion) the number of casualties may exceed the capacity of the medical and rescue services.

Triage with mass casualties

In an accident or natural disaster with mass casualties, the triage officer may have to make a choice between whom to save and whom to leave, possibly to die. This task is most appropriately performed by an experienced medical practitioner.

In such a situation, the principles of triage remain the same. However, order of priority may be 'reversed'. Priority may be given to casualties whose injuries can be rapidly treated with a good chance of permanent recovery rather than to those whose injuries would be time-consuming to treat and probably result in permanent disability.

For example, a casualty with a fractured spine would generally have a lower priority than one with internal abdominal bleeding. The latter will probably fully recover with immediate hospital treatment but may die if treatment is left for an hour or so, whereas the former will probably result in permanent paralysis whether treatment is given straight away or in a few hours.

The safe environment

Making your environment safe will help prevent many accidents. It can save lives. Every first aider has a role to promote 'preventive first aid'.

Remember, young children do not have a fully developed sense of danger. They are inquisitive, like to explore and are adventurous whether in the home or outdoors. And they can be very quiet! As children cannot fully protect themselves, we as adults must do all we can to ensure a safe environment.

While many of the precautions outlined in this chapter are for child safety, we also have to ensure safety for ourselves and our community—at home, on the roads, in the workplace and outdoors.

Safety in the Home

Precautions in the home are necessary to ensure the safety of everyone. When there are young children in the home, extra precautions have to be taken. Teaching children safety measures gives them an awareness of dangers and of how to act safely.

External doors
- Keep front and back doors closed.
- Teach children not to open the door to strangers.
- Make sure door knobs and latches are out-of-reach of young children so they cannot get out without you knowing.
- Glass doors should be made of toughened or laminated glass, with motif or decals to ensure visibility.

Hallway
- Use rugs with non-slip backing to prevent tripping and falls.

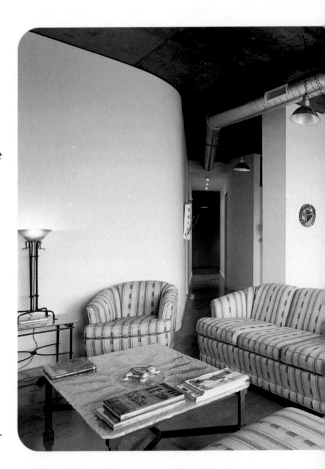

- Equip stairs with handrails.
- Ensure carpet on stairs is not loose.
- Keep halls and stairs free of toys.
- Don't let children play on public landings and stairs of unit blocks.
- Have stairways, corridors and dark areas well lit.

Family or lounge room
- Check for objects that may cause injury.
- Have a stable guard for fires and radiators.
- Keep scissors and sewing equipment out-of-reach of children.

- Use dummy plugs in power points (all rooms).

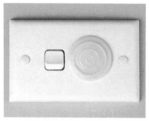

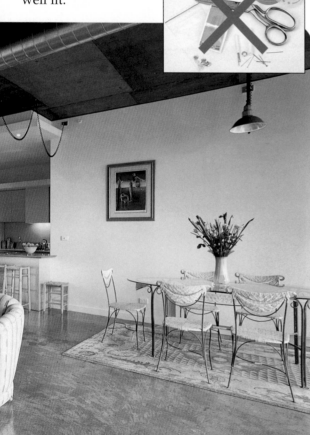

- Place trailing electrical cords out-of-reach of young children.
- Have eye level markings on glass doors and floor-to-ceiling windows.

Bedroom
- Do not smoke in bed.
- Have safety rails on top bunks.
- Keep perfume, hairspray, aftershave and makeup out-of-reach of children.
- Don't leave a glass within reach of children.

289

Kitchen
- Saucepan handles should be turned away from edge of stove.
- Keep electrical cords and hot food away from children's reach.
- Unplug appliances when not in use.

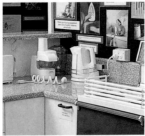

- Ensure electrical cords are not worn.
- Have electrical goods checked regularly for unsafe wear.
- Use safety-designed jugs, saucepans, electrical cords, stove guards.

- Store sharp knives safely.
- Store domestic cleaners safely.
- Store plastic bags safely.

- Fit cupboards with childproof locks.
- Use place mats in preference to a table-cloth (small children may pull anything on a cloth onto themselves).

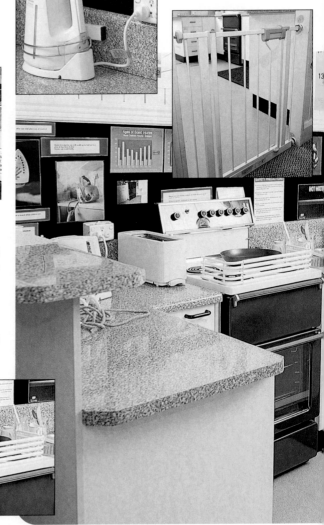

Bathroom
- Have a non-slip mat.
- Store medicines out-of-reach of children.
- Return unwanted medicines to your chemist.
- Set thermostat on water heater to around 50°C.

- Watch children in the bath.
- Do not allow electrical equipment in wet areas.
- Keep floor dry.
- Keep razor blades and shavers out-of-reach of children.

Laundry
- Store soaps, detergents and other cleaning products safely.
- Dry up spilt water.
- Have washing machines checked regularly, by a service tradesperson.

Other
- Store poisonous sub-stances out-of-reach of children.
- Store firearms safely and out-of-reach of children.
- Install smoke detec-tors on all levels; check regularly.
- Keep heating and cooling systems in good order.
- Have a fire extinguisher readily accessible.
- Have a torch and spare batteries.
- Don't leave bowls of pet food lying around.
- Have earth leakage detectors fitted (to prevent electrocu-tion).
- Keep a complete first aid kit.

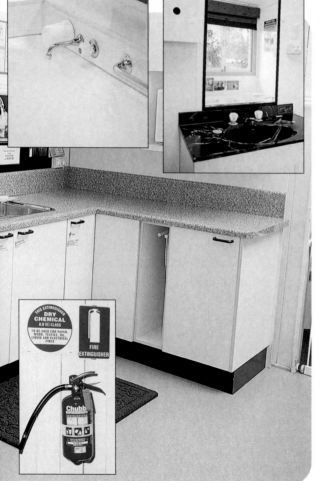

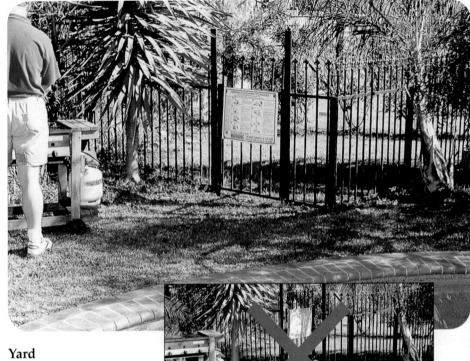

Yard

- Install a childproof fence around pool.
- Supervise children at all times when swimming.
- Cover pool vacuum area and enclose filter equipment.
- Have a non-slip surface around pool.
- Don't leave fires and BBQs unattended.
- Don't leave fuel and gas containers in the sun.
- Store chemicals safely.

- Keep firm lids on garbage bins.
- Wrap broken glass with thick layers of paper before placing in bin.
- Use a soft, level surface (e.g. woodchips) under swings and other play equipment.
- Teach children to use equipment properly.

- Ensure backyard is fenced off from road.
- Read safety directions before using fertilisers and poisons.
- Use eye-protection and adequate footwear when using lawnmower and other garden equipment.

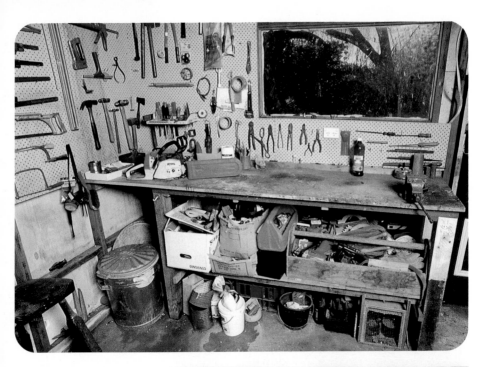

Shed

- Remove doors from old refrigerators.
- Don't place poisons in soft drink bottles.
- Label and store poisons (e.g. weed-killers, kerosene) safely.
- Use power tools in accordance with instructions.
- Store tools safely.
- Lock up firearms (unloaded and dismantled).

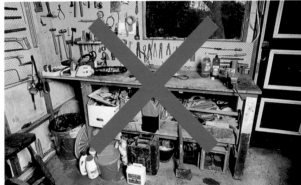

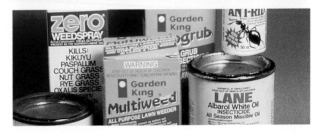

BABIES AND YOUNG CHILDREN

Some extra safety precautions have to be taken when there is a baby or a young child in the house. Babies and young children do not have a fully developed sense of danger. Young children are very curious and eager to explore their environment. If there are older children, care has to be taken with some of their toys which may be dangerous for babies and young children.

- Use a safety harness in a highchair.
- Use a playpen when necessary to keep baby safe.
- Don't leave baby unattended on a change table or bed.
- Make sure cot has sides.
- Do not use a pillow with children under 1 year (they could suffocate).
- Place baby on back or side to sleep, not face down.

Toys and clothing
- Clothing should be of non-flammable material.
- Clothing should be form-fitting if likely to be worn near open fires or radiators.
- Keep toys or other objects with small parts away from children (they could choke).
- Remove ribbons from a baby's soft toys.
- Make sure toys don't have sharp edges.
- Buy non-toxic paints and crayons.

Safety on the Road

- Wear seatbelts.
- Provide babies and young children with age/weight appropriate safety restraints.
- Always secure safety restraints correctly.
- Ensure car is roadworthy.
- Ensure children outside the car are in full view when you reverse the car.
- Ensure children are never left unattended in a car.
- Don't let a child play with car windows, whether manual or electric.
- Use child locks on rear doors with young children.
- Don't leave cigarettes, matches, or cigarette lighters in a car.
- Obey road signs and traffic laws.
- Don't drive if over blood alcohol limit.
- Bikes must have reflectors and lights.
- Wear bright clothes when riding a bike.
- Wear protective headgear and knee and elbow pads when skating or skateboarding.
- Wear helmet when riding a bicycle or motorbike.
- Hold a small child's hand when crossing road together.
- Always cross the road at a pedestrian crossing, a corner or traffic lights, or use an underpass or overpass.
- Carry a first aid kit in car and on extended bicycle rides.

SAFETY IN THE WORKPLACE

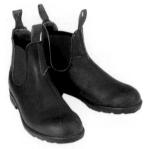

- Have adequate first aid supplies and be trained in their use.
- Wear appropriate protective gear—eyes, ears, mouth/nose, hands and feet.
- Know and follow safety rules.
- Use warning signs to mark danger areas and dangerous equipment.
- Have fire extinguishers readily accessible.
- Develop and practise an emergency evacuation plan.
- Floors should be clean with an even surface.
- NEVER tamper with or override safety devices on machinery.
- Ensure HAZCHEM signs are displayed when necessary.

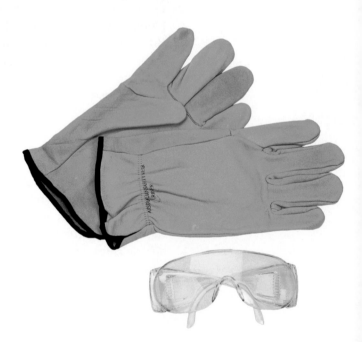

Safety Outdoors

SWIMMING

- Swim only on patrolled beaches, between the flags.
- Obey lifesavers' instructions.
- Avoid swimming in isolated rivers or dams unless accompanied by other people.
- Check water depth before diving into any water.
- Avoid diving in unknown rivers or dams.
- Avoid alcohol before swimming.
- Supervise children at all times near water.
- Do not get into a swimming hole unless there is a clear way out.

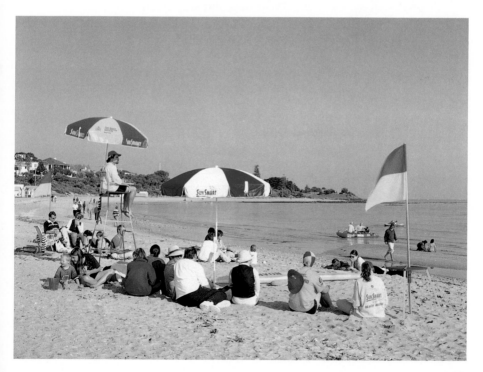

BOATING

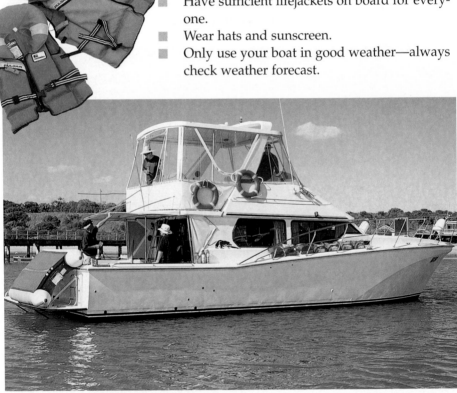

- Carry safety equipment and sufficient fuel and water.
- Always carry appropriate communication equipment.
- Know the distress signals and local regulations for boating.
- Ensure boat engine is in good working order before use.
- Ensure there are no petrol spills or leaks when boating.
- Always tell someone where you are going and what time you expect to be back.
- Always slow down near swimmers and small boats.
- Have sufficient lifejackets on board for everyone.
- Wear hats and sunscreen.
- Only use your boat in good weather—always check weather forecast.

IN THE BUSH

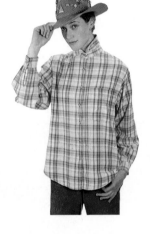

- Always hike or camp with companions.
- Inform someone about where you are going, and when you plan to arrive and return.
- Take water, adequate food, matches, compass and map of the area.
- Take mobile phone.
- Wait for help if lost and stay with companions.
- Label all dangerous items clearly.
- Make sure stoves and lanterns are safe.
- Ensure containers of hot food cannot be tipped over.
- Ensure collapsible tables and chairs are safe.
- Wear appropriate clothes and thick-soled shoes.
- Protect yourself against sunburn and insect bites.
- Make sure your camp fire is out before leaving.
- Know how to prevent and treat overexposure to heat or cold.
- Carry an appropriate first aid kit.

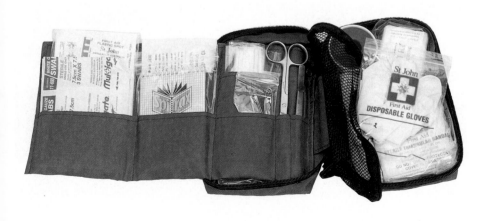

IN THE DESERT OR REMOTE AREA WILDERNESS

- Carry adequate supplies of water (at least 4 litres per person per day, stored in the shade).
- Rest in the shade of the vehicle and stay together if vehicle breaks down or you are lost.
- Wear hats, long sleeves and trousers and thick-soled boots.
- Take a CB radio, mobile phone or satellite phone for communication.
- Know how to lay adequate signals for rescuers.
- Tell authorities (e.g. rangers, police, station owners) where you are going and expected arrival times.

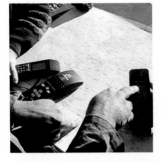

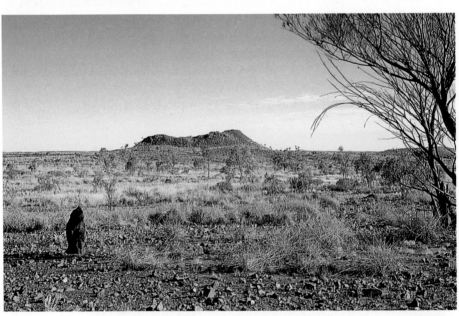

SAFETY AND FIRES

FIRE SAFETY RULES FOR THE HOME

1 Have the emergency telephone number handy—☎ *call 000.*

2 Have a fire extinguisher in a central place (not near the stove).

3 Have a fire blanket or woollen blanket in the kitchen (for use on burning oil).

4 Fit smoke detectors and check regularly.

5 Ensure electrical wiring and appliances are in good repair.

6 Keep flammable materials including matches and lighters safely.

7 Be aware of risks of falling asleep while smoking.

8 Do not fit security grilles to all windows and doors.

9 Develop and practise an evacuation procedure.

10 Teach children STOP DROP–ROLL *(see p. 215)* and GET DOWN LOW AND GO, GO, GO! (in case home is filled with smoke).

EVACUATION FROM A BURNING BUILDING

Fires can burn and spread very quickly in a building—even a minor fire can escalate in minutes to a serious blaze. Often smoke and fumes from the fire are more dangerous than the flames. It is easy to be overcome by smoke and a lack of oxygen. Furnishings containing synthetic materials give off toxic fumes when burning.

Panic is another danger which can spread very quickly. Therefore it is important to remain calm yourself and to calm anyone else involved.

IN CASE OF FIRE (HOME OR OTHER BUILDING)

1 Remain calm.

2 ☎ *Call 000 for emergency services* (from a place outside building if necessary).

3 Activate any fire alarms.

4 Extinguish fire if possible.

If it becomes necessary to leave building:

5 Shut doors and windows to contain fire.

6 Carry out evacuation procedure.

7 Leave the building quickly without running.

8 Turn off power if possible.

9 **DO NOT** go back inside for anything.

A fire in a large building (e.g. hotel, office block) can be extremely dangerous and knowing how to get out could mean the difference between life and death. When you first go into an unfamiliar building, check where the fire exits and the fire extinguishers are located. If you have to be evacuated, follow the instructions of those organising evacuation.

FIRE IN A LARGE BUILDING—ADDITIONAL POINTS

1 **DO NOT** use lifts under any circumstances.

2 **DO NOT** open a door if it feels hot.

3 If unable to get to fire exit, return to your room:
   - stuff wet towels and cloths over any cracks (e.g. under doors and windows) and vents
   - turn off ventilation system (if possible)
   - call the front desk or emergency services to report the fire and your location.

4 **DO NOT** enter a burning building—leave it to emergency services.

5 If overhead high voltage lines are involved, wait for electricity authorities; direct others away.

6 If casualties are affected by any of the following, move them to fresh air—asphyxia (lack of oxygen); carbon monoxide poisoning; poisoning from toxic fumes; irritation of respiratory tract and eyes.

BUSHFIRES

Note: Anyone in or near bushfire prone areas should familiarise themselves with local guidelines and recommendations.

Not only people who live in rural areas are at risk of bushfires in Australia. Even if you live in a city, you may still be at risk. There are a number of long-term measures you can take to protect your home.

▶ Clear a fuel break of about 30–40 metres around the home.

▶ Make sure gutters are clear of leaves and other vegetation.

▶ Clear undergrowth, overhanging branches and any flammable material and liquids from around the house.

- Fit windows, vents, chimneys and doors with screens to stop sparks entering.
- Seal off area under house.
- Ensure access to your own emergency water supply (there may be no mains pressure).
- **PLAN IN ADVANCE** whether to stay or evacuate in case of fire.
- Have an emergency kit prepared (heavy cotton clothing including long-sleeved top and long trousers, leather shoes and gloves, face covering, torches, bottles of water).
- If relevant, know where your evacuation centre is.

When a bushfire is in the vicinity of your home, there are further measures you can take:

- Put on clothing from emergency kit.
- Carry out your plan; if evacuating **LEAVE EARLY** (take pets).
- Plug downpipes with sand- or earth-filled bags.
- Fill gutters with water.
- Hose those parts of the building where fire could take hold.
- Dampen the ground around the house.
- Put wet, rolled towels under doors and around windows.
- Close windows.
- Place furniture away from windows.
- Secure pets in house if you haven't evacuated.

Wet towels and woollen or cotton blankets can be used for personal protection against fire and to minimise smoke inhalation.

First aid in the workplace

The responsibility of ensuring workplace safety rests with all employers and employees. All workplaces have hazards, which may or may not be obvious. They may include aspects of the physical environment, materials and equipment used, and work practices.

Each State and Territory has a number of Acts, Regulations and Ordinances which regulate the work environment and provide minimum standards for the protection of workers' health and safety.

The role of the first aider in assisting with ongoing safety of workers and in managing injuries and illnesses is outlined in this chapter. Some legal responsibilities of employers, employees and the first aider are also discussed.

FIRST AID IN THE WORKPLACE

First aider's responsibilities

The main role of the first aider in the workplace is to provide first aid management of illness and injury. Other responsibilities include:

- record keeping
- recognition and reporting of health and safety hazards
- participation in safety programs
- maintenance of a first aid kit and/or first aid room

Prevention of injury and illness should be of the utmost importance in every workplace. Injuries can cause much trauma and cost time and money. Unsafe working conditions lead to inefficiencies in production. Preventive first aid is a major part of the first aider's responsibilities.

Ongoing safety education is crucial for the prevention of accidents. Working according to safe-practice guidelines has proven to be efficient in the long-term.

All workplaces have hazards. Chemicals, plant and machinery, tools and equipment, material handling and storage, electrical installations and radiation are obvious dangers. In workplaces such as offices, the dangers are not as obvious.

TYPES OF INJURY IN THE WORKPLACE

Back injuries comprise approximately one quarter of all injuries in the workplace and are the most frequently reported result of industrial accidents. Such injuries cause much physical suffering to the employee and cost employers millions of dollars in lost time and medical expenses.

Skin rashes, **skin infections** and **allergic reactions** to substances are also commonly reported in the workplace and comprise about 50% of occupational disease. Various chemicals and other agents and hot, humid work conditions are common causes of rashes, allergic reactions and skin infections.

Contact dermatitis is one of the two main types of occupational skin rash and may be caused by:
▶ physical irritants (e.g. friction, heat, moisture, ultraviolet light)
▶ chemical irritants (e.g. acids, alkalis, mercury compounds)
▶ fat solvents (e.g. thinners, formaldehyde)

Allergic dermatitis is the other main skin disease resulting from workplace conditions. It may result from a sensitivity to oils and coal tars, rubber, dyes, resins and plastics, and even soaps and cosmetics.

Skin infections are caused by bacteria (e.g. *staphylococcus aureus* or golden staph) and fungi (e.g. tinea). Fungal infections are more common in hot, humid workplaces.

Radiation burns may be caused by the sun, welding arcs, ultraviolet rays or nuclear accidents. Extensive superficial burns and blisters can result. Nuclear irradiation can also severely damage internal organs with consequences such as diarrhoea, vomiting and shock. Death may occur even after twenty-four hours.

Hearing damage can occur in workplaces where there is exposure to constant and/or a higher than normal level of noise. Most States in Australia have legislation aimed at preserving the hearing of people working in such conditions and requiring use of protective devices.

Chest and blast injuries and amputation are likely to occur in particular types of workplaces and usually result from accidents associated with heavy equipment and machinery.

Accidents with chemicals usually occur in the workplace because of a lack of awareness of necessary precautions. First aiders should be familiar with chemicals used in the workplace, the potential hazards and appropriate first aid management. They should understand work processes to enable recognition of possible harmful emissions.

In the **office environment**, awareness of fire evacuation procedures and the location of the nearest fire extinguisher and first aid kit is essential.

LEGAL ISSUES

State requirements

Legislation covering safety requirements in the workplace varies from State to State and from industry to industry. Each State and Territory has an Occupational and Workplace Health and Safety Act and a number of other Acts, Ordinances and Regulations providing a set of minimum standards.

Legal issues arising in first aid in the workplace include:
- consent to treatment—a rational casualty can refuse first aid
- respect for casualty's privacy

▶ confidentiality of records
▶ destruction of records
▶ liability for improper or negligent administration of first aid

Consent to first aid treatment

As a general rule, mentally competent adults have the right to refuse any treatment, even if that treatment is necessary to save their lives. Treatment given to a person without consent may constitute an assault.

Consent can be implied or expressed. If the casualty goes to the first aid room and cooperates with the first aid officer, consent is *implied* (taken as given). Consent is *expressed* when oral or written permission is given.

In some situations a person cannot give consent to treatment—for example, if the injury or illness has affected the ability to make an informed choice, if the casualty is unconscious, or is very young or mentally disabled. In these cases, consent is not required and a qualified person may administer any necessary treatment to save the person's life or to prevent serious illness or further injury.

Privacy and confidentiality

Legislation varies with respect to who can have access to first aid records, the extent of this access, and what incidents have to be reported. However, the following people have the right to access:
▶ ambulance officers or a treating doctor
▶ those investigating workplace illness or injury (police, coroner, workplace inspection authority, the courts)
▶ employer (e.g. to ensure injury was work-related or to assist in identifying cause)

With the casualty's agreement, access is given to:

▶   insurance company handling claim
▶   union representatives or occupational health and safety committees

Legislation also requires that occupational incidents causing serious injury or death must be reported to the relevant government authority. Legislation may require the employer to report the incident, but the first aider to complete required notification.

Despite legitimate access by many people to first aid records, the privacy of the casualty should be respected to the greatest extent possible. The person controlling the records has a responsibility to ensure they are only released to people with appropriate authority. The casualty should be informed if access has been given. A record should be kept of who has had access to particular documents, and when and why.

Destruction of records   There are no general rules regarding destruction of records. Some legislation specifies how long records should be kept. Considerations include the limitations period after which cases cannot be brought to court, and the period during which compensation claims can be made. In general, casualty records should be kept for at least seven years.

Liability   First aiders are only liable for any injury caused by them if negligence can be shown. The person suing must be able to show, among other things, a duty of care, and that the treatment was not reasonable in the circumstances.

Protection against legal liability is afforded if treatment is in accordance with a St John

Ambulance Australia first aid manual and within the first aider's level of training, if complete and legible records are maintained, and if skills are maintained and updated.

FIRST AID ROOMS AND KITS

The relevant Acts set out minimum requirements for availability and contents of first aid rooms and kits. Extra equipment will vary according to hazards associated with specific workplaces and industries.

First aid rooms

Guidelines laid down by the National Health and Medical Research Council (NHMRC) state that first aid rooms should have:

- minimum floor area of 15 square metres
- good illumination and ventilation
- easy access to toilets
- access door at least 1.2 metres wide
- hot and cold running water
- adequate space for rendering first aid

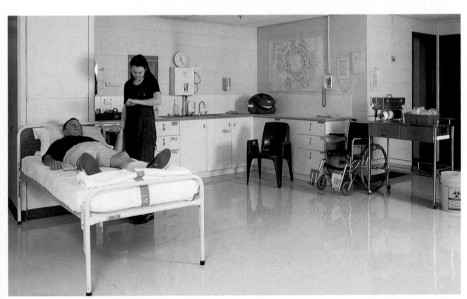

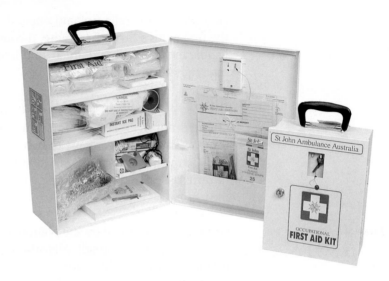

First aid kits

A first aid kit should be readily accessible to all those in the workplace. It should be made of metal, be lockable, dust and moisture proof, and large enough to store all first aid requirements. It should be clearly marked with a white cross on a green background and contain first aid instructions.

First aid kits and rooms must be stocked with supplies appropriate for managing injuries that may occur in the workplace, and all equipment must be maintained for operational readiness.

A notice giving the name and location of the person responsible for first aid should be placed on the kit or outside the first aid room. The first aider has the responsibility to ensure that:

▶ the first aid room is kept tidy and clean
▶ first aid stock is regularly checked and replenished
▶ medication is clearly labelled and stored as directed
▶ expiry dates are checked regularly

Reporting Illness and Injury

The majority of Acts require deaths and various classes of accidents to be reported to the appropriate government authority. First aiders should be aware of the documentation requirements of the Acts, Ordinances and Regulations relevant to their workplace.

NEED FOR RECORDS

Documentation

Employers are required to maintain a written record of all injuries and illnesses at the place of employment. Legislation may require that work-related injuries and illnesses are recorded on an accident report form *(see p. 315)* and in an accident register.

Accurate reporting and documentation of casualty information are important functions of the first aider. This applies to all incidents where workers seek advice or treatment relating to first aid. Maintenance of good, accurate records is necessary:

- ▶ for proper clinical management
- ▶ as the law requires such records
- ▶ to protect the first aider against possible litigation and prosecution
- ▶ to protect individuals if controversy ensues
- ▶ to protect the company
- ▶ to provide information for evaluation of injury and illness trends

FIRST AID RECORD KEEPING

Documentation must be accurate and legible. It should include the employee's factual account of the incident, but not opinion and hearsay.

Records should be written at the time treatment is given or as soon afterwards as possible. They must be written in ink or ballpoint and never erased. Mistakes have to be crossed through and 'wrong entry' written next to them. Records of accidents should be validated and signed by the employee involved.

All medical records must be kept strictly confidential and should:

▶ be stored in a locked cupboard

▶ be accessible only to first aiders and authorised personnel

▶ not be made available to unauthorised personnel

TYPES OF RECORDS

The format of records varies between industries and between workplaces because of different policy requirements and legislation.

Referral letters

Where employees are referred to a doctor or hospital, referral letters should accompany them giving:

▶ brief personal details (name, date of birth, address, job, allergies, previous medical history)

▶ date

▶ history of injury/illness (what happened, when and where)

▶ observations (what seen/felt) and vital signs

▶ first aider's assessment of injury/illness

▶ first aid management (wound dressings, medication, referral)

▶ signature and status of first aider

If a chemical or toxic substance has been involved, all information should accompany the casualty to the doctor or hospital.

CONFIDENTIAL   **OB12**

Casualty Report

St John Ambulance Australia

Date	Duty			Member No.	Time in

Casualty Name	Surname	Given Names		Sex	D.O.B.

Casualty Address			Postcode	Telephone	Category

History	**Allergies** (list, if any)	☐ English speaking	☐ Non-English speaking
What			
How			
When			

Past Medical History:

☐ Not known	☐ Diabetes	☐ Epilepsy	☐ Medic Alert
☐ Nil	☐ Asthma	☐ Loss of Consciousness	☐ Hypertension
☐ Other:	☐ Cardiac	☐ Medication........................	

Casualty Assessment

Breathing [1]	Skin [2]	Pulse [3]	Conscious [4]	Other Signs & Symptoms
1. Unremarkable	1. Unremarkable	1. Unremarkable	1. Alert	
	2. Pale	2. Slow	2. Confused	
2. Shallow	3. Flushed	3. Rapid	3. Drowsy	
3. Absent	4. Moist/clammy	4. Strong	4. Unconscious	
4. Wheeze	5. Dry	5. Weak		
5. Gasping	6. Sweaty	6. Impalpable		
6. Rapid	7. Cool/Cold	7. Regular	**Overall Assessment:**	
7. Slow	8. Warm/Hot	8. Irregular		

Time	Pulse	Resp.	Temp.	Conscious State				Pupils' size	Pupils' reaction		Other Observations
				E	V	M	TOTAL	R | L	R	L	

		Location [5]	RICE [6]	Slings [7]	Dressing [8]
	A - Abrasion	1. Head	1. Rest	1. Collar & Cuff	1. Transparent
	Bl - Bleeding	2. Facial	2. Ice	2. St John	2. Adhesive strips
	Bu - Burns	3. Chest	Time on:	3. Triangular	3. Dry dressing
	C - Contusion	4. Abdomen	3. Compression	4. Comp. bandage	4. Non adherent
	D - Deformity	5. Limb	4. Elevation	Time applied:	5. Other
	F - ? Fracture	6. Spinal	5. All of above		
	L - Laceration	7. Multiple	**Posture** [9]	**Oxygen** [10]	**Referred to** [11]
	P - Pain	8. Back	1. Legs up	1. Mask	1. Hosp. (AMB.)
	S - Swelling		2. Coma	2. Demand valve	2. Hosp. (CAR)
	T - Tenderness		3. Sitting	3. Nasal prongs	3. Own doctor
			4. Lying	Litres per min.	4. Nil
				4. Assisted vent.	Discharge advice ☐

Treatment:

Medication Given: Dose   Time Given

Medication with Casualty	Yes ☐ No ☐	Refused Treatment ☐	Witness
Signature:	Print Name	Division:	
Top copy to District/Division	Pink copy with Casualty	Yellow copy to Member	Time Out

ST JOHN AMBULANCE AUSTRALIA CASUALTY REPORT

Injury report

An injury report is a full account of what happened as related by the casualty. It should have sufficient information to satisfy statutory requirements, (*see p. 315* for sample St John form). A copy of this report is given to the supervisor and safety officer.

Daily attendance register

A first aider should also maintain a daily attendance register. This contains a summary of all casualties seen during each shift, each entry being signed by the first aider. This register may be perused in court, sometimes years after an initial injury or illness.

Injury statistics

Injury statistics are a summary of illnesses and injuries occurring in a workplace over a given time. Statistics are useful in detecting trends and can be used to prevent accidents, reduce their severity, and evaluate safety procedures.

More detailed information on first aid in the workplace can be found in *Occupational First Aid* (published by St John Ambulance Australia).

19

Respiratory emergencies

Severe or continued difficulty with breathing is referred to as respiratory distress, an emergency condition requiring immediate attention.

Respiratory distress can be caused by an injury or illness that results in insufficient oxygen in the blood. As a result the casualty gasps for air and may breathe faster.

A drug overdose can also lead to respiratory failure, but in this situation the casualty's breathing is usually laboured and uneven, and may become slower and finally stop.

This chapter discusses the causes and management of respiratory emergencies. It also highlights ways in which choking, a common cause of respiratory distress, can be avoided in both adults and children.

RESPIRATORY SYSTEM

Oxygen is vital to life. In breathing, four of the body's systems have to work together. The **respiratory system** ensures oxygen is taken into the body; the **circulatory system** ensures it is transported to all parts of the body; and the **nervous system** ensures the correct messages are transmitted to the **musculoskeletal system**, so it can perform the movements necessary for breathing.

Injuries and illnesses can affect these systems and impair breathing. Injury to the area of the brain which controls breathing may impair or stop breathing. If the heart stops beating, blood is no longer pumped through the body and the casualty will stop breathing.

MECHANICS OF BREATHING

Oxygen and carbon dioxide are exchanged in the lungs via the thin walls of the alveoli and their capillaries. The oxygen taken up by the blood is then transported to all parts of the body. The blood also brings carbon dioxide and other waste products from around the body to the lungs where they enter the alveoli and are expelled from the body on exhalation.

The brain automatically monitors the amount of oxygen and carbon dioxide in the blood and responds to the levels by changing the rate and depth of breathing.

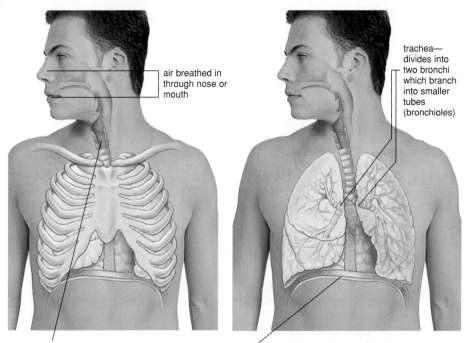

air breathed in through nose or mouth

trachea—divides into two bronchi which branch into smaller tubes (bronchioles)

air transferred to lungs via trachea (windpipe)

diaphragm—a large muscle which expands chest to pull air into lungs; as it relaxes, air is forced out

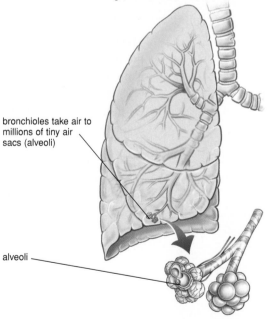

bronchioles take air to millions of tiny air sacs (alveoli)

alveoli

Mechanics of breathing

Normal–abnormal respirations

When a person is breathing normally, the body receives as much oxygen as it needs to function properly. When the body is not getting sufficient oxygen the person will have signs of respiratory distress.

The rate, rhythm and depth of breathing are all used to assess breathing. The **rate** is the number of times a person breathes in and out in one minute. The normal rate will vary for infants, children, and adults. A breathing rate that is too slow or too fast is a sign of an emergency.

BREATHING RATES AT REST—BREATHS PER MINUTE

Age group	Range of normal rates	Too slow	Too fast
infant (under 1 yr)	30–50	below 25	above 60
young child (1–8 yrs)	20–30	below 15	above 40
child (over 8 yrs)/adult	10–20	below 10	above 30

The breathing **rhythm** refers to the regularity of the time interval between breaths. When a person is breathing normally, the intervals are even and breathing appears effortless. Irregular breathing, with uneven intervals, can indicate a respiratory disorder.

The breathing **depth** refers to the amount of air the person breathes in, in one breathing cycle—doctors call this the 'tidal volume'.

RESPIRATORY EMERGENCIES

> **Warning**
>
> Respiratory distress is a life-threatening emergency. Recognition of early signs and symptoms is more important than knowing the specific cause.
> Adequate care can be given without knowing the actual cause.

Signs and symptoms

▶ breathing is:
  - too fast or too slow
  - irregular
  - too shallow or too deep
  - noisy or rasping

▶ person is:
  - struggling or gasping for air
  - becoming tired from trying to breathe
  - semi-conscious

▶ may feel dizzy or out of breath and show signs of anxiety

▶ lips, ears and fingernails bluish

▶ abnormal chest movement

▶ air cannot be felt moving out of mouth or nose

CAUSES OF RESPIRATORY EMERGENCIES

Respiratory distress can be caused by an injury such as a broken rib, by an induced condition such as hyperventilation, by poisoning such as capsicum spray exposure or by an illness such as asthma. It can also be the first sign of other serious respiratory emergencies or even of a heart attack.

CAUSES OF A RESPIRATORY EMERGENCY

Injuries	Illnesses	Poisoning	Other conditions
• broken ribs	• asthma	• inhaled poison	• hyperventilation
• near drowning	• stroke	e.g. carbon	• airway obstruction
• knife or gun-	• allergic reaction	monoxide	• choking
shot wound	• pneumonia	• injected poison	• emotional stress
• burns to the	• congestive	e.g. blue-ringed	• suffocation
face	heart failure	octopus	• strangulation
• head injury	• emphysema	• smoke or	• hanging
• chest is	• respiratory	gas inhalation	
compressed	infections	• toxic fumes	
and cannot	• heart attack	• drug or medication	
expand and		overdose	
contract		e.g. heroin,	
• electrical		sleeping tablets	
injuries		• capsicum spray	

Respiratory distress can lead to respiratory arrest and death. Respiratory arrest (cessation of breathing), means the body is no longer receiving the oxygen it requires to keep functioning. After 3–4 minutes without oxygen, the body's systems begin to fail—the heart stops pumping blood and the circulatory system stops functioning. All other systems start to close down.

MANAGEMENT OF RESPIRATORY EMERGENCIES

CHOKING (AIRWAY OBSTRUCTION)

A person chokes when the airway is partly or completely blocked. The casualty usually has trouble breathing and, if obstruction is complete, cannot breathe at all. Unless given first aid, the casualty may die. The first aider's aim is to dislodge the object stuck in the throat, to clear the casualty's airway.

Signs and symptoms

- ▶ clutching the throat
- ▶ coughing, wheezing, gagging
- ▶ difficulty speaking or swallowing
- ▶ making violent attempts to breathe
- ▶ face, neck, lips, ears, fingernails turning blue
- ▶ making a whistling or 'crowing' noise
- ▶ collapsing or becoming unconscious

CAUSES OF CHOKING

Foreign objects	Unconsciousness	Injury or illness
• eating or drinking too quickly • swallowing small bones • not chewing food sufficiently • tablets or capsules	• tongue falls to back of throat if casualty on back • saliva, blood or vomit in throat	• injury to throat causes swelling of airway • illness causes swelling e.g. asthma, allergic reaction

Note: Children are particularly vulnerable to choking on small objects (e.g. toys, buttons, coins, peanuts).

MANAGEMENT OF CHOKING—ADULTS *

Partial blockage

1 Encourage casualty to relax and breathe deeply.

2 Ask casualty to cough (to remove object).

3 If unsuccessful, bend casualty well forward.

4 Give 4 sharp blows between shoulder-blades.

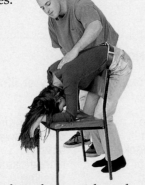

5 If blockage has not cleared, place casualty on side on floor.

6 ☎ *Call 000 for an ambulance.*

Total blockage

1 Bend casualty forward from the waist and give 4 sharp blows between shoulderblades.

2 If unsuccessful, lie casualty on side on floor.

3 Give lateral chest thrusts by placing your hands on the side of casualty's chest below armpit and giving 4 quick down-ward thrusts.

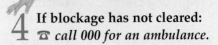

4 **If blockage has not cleared:** ☎ *call 000 for an ambulance.*

5 Repeat steps until help arrives or blockage clears.

6 Follow DRABC. **DRABC** ➤

For management of choking in children see page 58.

SMOKE AND GAS INHALATION

Inhalation of smoke, gas or toxic fumes can cause a respiratory emergency. A flue leak (e.g. from a stove, heater) can cause the carbon monoxide level in a room to become dangerously high. Inhalation of smoke can reduce the amount of oxygen getting to the lungs and also cause swelling and burning of the airway. The casualty may inhale dangerous levels of toxic fumes (e.g. from paint, thinners, petroleum products and adhesives), especially in confined or insufficiently ventilated spaces. This can result in unconsciousness and death. **An inhalation injury is always considered a life-threatening emergency. It is important to ensure the casualty gets medical help as quickly as possible.**

Warning
It may be some hours before the effect of inhaling toxic fumes interferes with a person's breathing.

MANAGEMENT OF INHALATION EMERGENCY

1 Follow DRABC. **DRABC**

2 Remove casualty from smoke or toxic atmosphere—if safe.

3 Sit casualty upright.

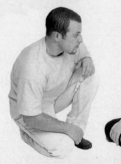

4 Loosen tight clothing.

6 If breathing ceases, give EAR.

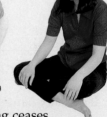

5 Ensure plenty of fresh air.

7 ☎ *Call 000 for an ambulance.*

HYPERVENTILATION

Hyperventilation is a result of involuntary over-breathing. It can be due to excitement, hysteria, stress or other emotion. Rate and depth of breathing are more than is necessary to maintain normal levels of carbon dioxide in the blood. Consequently, carbon dioxide in the blood falls, causing a range of symptoms. Signs may include shallow, rapid breathing, rapid pulse, feeling of suffocating, dizziness, pins and needles, tingling or spasms of hands and feet.

MANAGEMENT OF EMOTIVE HYPERVENTILATION

1 Follow DRABC.

2 Calm casualty; remove to a quiet, private place.

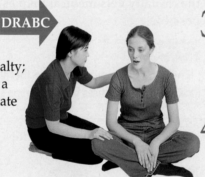

3 Encourage slow, regular breathing—slowly count breaths aloud.

4 Seek medical aid.

STRANGULATION

The casualty may be conscious or unconscious.

MANAGEMENT OF STRANGULATION/HANGING

1 If casualty hanging, support weight of body.

2 Remove any constricting material/free neck from noose.

3 Follow DRABC.

4 ☎ *Call 000 for an ambulance.*

NEAR DROWNING

In near drowning, a person gasping for air while trying to stay afloat may inhale only a small amount of water. The casualty usually has little water in the lungs because the muscles of the larynx (voice box) close the airway to stop water entering. However, the spasm which prevents water going in also prevents air from going in. Mucous plugs form. As a result, the casualty suffocates and becomes unconscious. **Every second is vital in management of near drowning.**

> ### Warning
>
> **DO NOT** attempt a rescue if you think you may not have the swimming ability or strength required to complete the rescue.

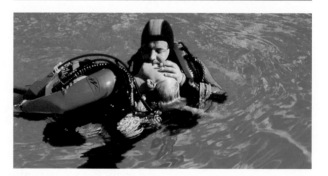

MANAGEMENT OF NEAR DROWNING

1 Follow DRABC. **DRABC**

2 Check and clear airway.

3 Begin EAR as soon as possible (in water if necessary).

4 Check pulse—if absent begin CPR.

5 ☎ *Call 000 for an ambulance.*

SWOLLEN THROAT TISSUES

Throat tissues can swell as a result of injury, allergic reaction (to bites, stings, food etc.), infection, burns, and inhalation of hot gases. When the throat becomes swollen, breathing is difficult.

MANAGEMENT OF SWOLLEN THROAT TISSUES

1 Follow DRABC. DRABC

2 If casualty has medication (e.g. for known allergy), ensure it is taken.

3 Apply a cold compress to the throat.

4 If breathing ceases, give EAR.

5 ☎ *Call 000 for an ambulance.*

CAPSICUM SPRAY EXPOSURE

Capsicum spray is available in a number of commercial forms and is being used more commonly by police forces all over Australia to subdue aggressive people. It is carried in a spray can and regarded as an offensive weapon. When used as a weapon, the spray is aimed at the face. The active agent can be absorbed by the mouth, nose, eyes and across intact skin—without damage to tissue. While it is intended that only the aggressor will be affected, without taking care, police, bystanders and first aiders may also be affected.

Exposure to the spray causes intense pain, spasm of eyelids and wheeziness (usually in a person prone to asthma). These symptoms will incapacitate most people exposed to the spray.

MANAGEMENT OF CASUALTY SPRAYED WITH CAPSICUM

1   Follow DRABC. **DRABC**▶

2   Protect your body, hands and eyes as much as possible using goggles, gloves and clothing.

3   Absorb excess capsicum solution with paper towel or similar and dispose of thoughtfully.

4   If casualty is cooperative, move to fresh air and place in a comfortable sitting position. If this is not possible, ventilate the room.

5   Check airway and breathing—if possible give 8–15 lpm of oxygen.

6   If casualty has breathing difficulty, use reliever puffer—as for management of asthma *(see p. 179)*

7   Wash exposed areas for 20 minutes with copious quantities of cool tap water—the used water must drain into a waste disposal system.

8   Wash eyes with water at room temperature for at least 15 minutes.

9   If affected area is below neck—an ice pack may be applied for 15 minutes about every 10 minutes to give relief.

10   Seek medical aid.

Note: The person may still be very violent and uncontrolled. There may also be excess spray on the casualty, their handlers, in the air and room and on flat surfaces, floor or ground. Ensure that police are still close by and you have a secure escape route or 'back away' area.

FOCUS ON SAFETY
PREVENTING RESPIRATORY EMERGENCIES IN ADULTS

Food
- cut into small pieces
- take small mouthfuls
- don't talk, laugh or gulp drinks with food in your mouth

Alcohol
- Drink in moderation

Vomiting
- lie casualty on side so there is less change of choking on vomit

Swimming
- swim only on patrolled beaches, between the flags
- avoid swimming in isolated rivers or dams unless accompanied by other people and a competent swimmer
- avoid alcohol before swimming
- check water depth before diving into any water
- avoid swimming in cold water for long periods

Water rescue
- only attempt a water rescue if you are a strong swimmer, and the water is not too deep for you

Inhalation
- wear breathing apparatus if you are likely to be exposed to toxic fumes
- avoid exposure to toxic fumes e.g. paint, thinners, petroleum products and adhesives

Drug or medication overdose
- make sure you follow the directions on medication packets correctly
- ensure that medications are contained in their original container
- avoid using or accepting social drugs

Advanced resuscitation

This chapter discusses two-person cardiopulmonary resuscitation (CPR) and defibrillation, which are advanced techniques for managing casualties requiring cardiopulmonary resuscitation.

Oxygen therapy is also used in cardiopulmonary resuscitation, and in treatment of other sick or injured casualties.

Two first aiders who are trained in two-person CPR may be at an accident scene. Two-person CPR, when performed in a rhythmical and synchronised manner, can be more effective than CPR performed by only one first aider and is less exhausting.

Extra oxygen can be useful in managing sick or injured casualties. However, oxygen may be administered only when the first aider is trained to administer it safely and knows the simple safety rules and regulations for storage of oxygen. This chapter also outlines the equipment used to administer extra oxygen.

Defibrillation involves giving a controlled shock to the heart, administered by trained personnel using specialised equipment.

TWO-PERSON CPR

When there are two first aiders at an emergency where CPR is required, one first aider can perform external chest compressions (ECC), while the other performs expired air resuscitation (EAR). However, two-person CPR (ECC+EAR) requires specific training. It is performed on adults and older children but not normally on small children because of their size.

Note: The more experienced first aider should perform EAR.

To be effective, two-person CPR has to be performed rhythmically so there is no noticeable break between the two actions. One breath is given after every 5 compressions (between 5th and 6th compressions). If the person giving the compressions counts aloud, for example in cycles from 1–5, the second first aider should be able to synchronise the breaths with the rhythm established by the compressions.

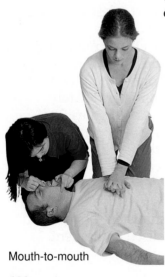

Mouth-to-mouth

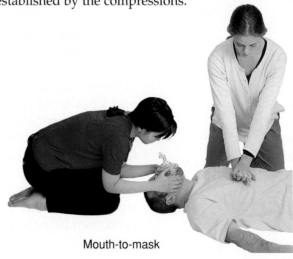

Mouth-to-mask

Note: The first aider giving the compressions DOES NOT STOP to allow for the breath to be given. The breath is given between every 5th and 6th compression.

The first aider giving breaths should also check for a pulse approximately every minute.

Note: The first aider giving the compressions MUST STOP during the pulse check.

MANAGEMENT OF TWO-PERSON CPR

1 Follow DRABC.

2 **First Aider 1:** Give 5 compressions.

3 **First Aider 2:** Give 1 effective breath between 5th and 6th compressions. (First Aider 1 does not stop compressions.)

4 Continue compressions and breaths in a ratio of 5:1. Compressions are given at a rate of about 100 a minute.

5 Continue resuscitation until:
- casualty shows signs of life
- qualified help arrives
- you both become exhausted.

6 Check pulse regularly (about every minute). Stop compressions for pulse check.

7 If pulse has returned, stop compressions but continue EAR until casualty resumes breathing unaided or ambulance personnel take over.

8 If breathing has resumed, place casualty in recovery position.

USE OF OXYGEN IN FIRST AID

WHEN TO ADMINISTER OXYGEN

Oxygen should be given to all people suffering from a lack of oxygen (hypoxia) due to an injury, or medical condition. It is used to assist in the resuscitation of a non-breathing casualty and as therapy for a breathing casualty (e.g. someone with smoke inhalation, or asthma). Conditions for which a casualty may require oxygen include:

- unconsciousness
- shock
- head injuries
- heart attack and heart conditions
- severe injury of any type
- heatstroke
- respiratory distress
- poisoning
- gas, smoke or capsicum spray inhalation
- chest conditions (casualty not able to breathe deeply enough, and thus at risk of hypoxia)
- abdominal injuries
- eye injuries (deterioration can occur very rapidly without oxygen)
- all other injuries—helps to reduce the extent of tissue damage as a result of insufficient oxygen

However, caution should be used in administering oxygen to a casualty who has chronic airway disease (e.g. severe emphysema, chronic bronchitis).

Oxygen may be administered to a breathing casualty by:

▶ face mask

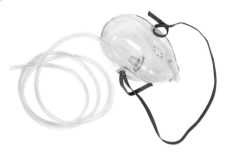

▶ nasal prongs (nasal cannula)

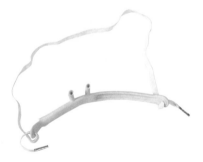

Oxygen may be administered to a non-breathing casualty by:

▶ mouth-to-mask with added oxygen

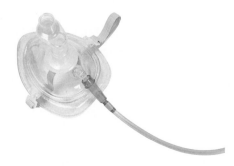

▶ oxygen-powered resuscitation

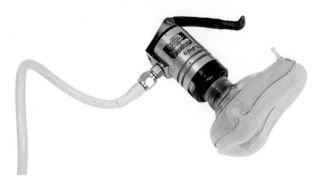

▶ bag-valve-mask system, soft bag

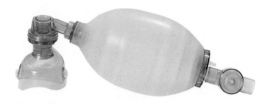

▶ bag-valve-mask system, self-inflating bag
with added oxygen

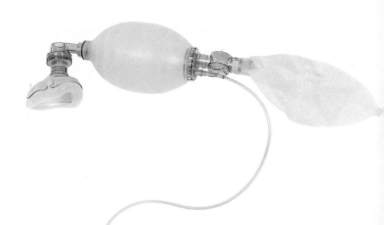

Oxygen should not be used if:
- ▶ there is any danger of fire
- ▶ first aider is not suitably qualified to use the equipment available

Note: If equipment is not immediately available, start EAR.

There are strict regulations concerning the safe storage and use of oxygen. Oxygen cylinders are filled and stored under high pressure and, as oxygen aids combustion, it is important to follow the safety precautions for its use.

Note: There is a high risk of combustion when oxygen is used in conjunction with oil or grease. Consequently, oil or grease MUST NOT be used on oxygen equipment.

CARE AND USE OF OXYGEN CYLINDERS

Selecting and 'cracking' oxygen cylinder

1 Select an appropriate size medical oxygen cylinder to suit apparatus to be used. Only medical oxygen, which is filtered and purified when cylinder filled, should be used (except in extreme emergency, *see p. 340*). (Medical oxygen cylinders are normally black with white around cylinder's neck or shoulder.)

2 Select a full cylinder, ensuring that a plastic dust seal is in place over the oxygen outlet hole. Leave seal in place until oxygen cylinder is required.

The seal, which usually also covers the indexing pin holes, enables the first aider to readily distinguish full cylinders from used ones.

The most commonly used oxygen cylinders are:

▶ C size cylinders = 400 to 490 litres of useable oxygen
▶ D size cylinders = 1640 litres of useable oxygen
▶ Special cylinders = approximately 200 litres of useable oxygen

'Portable' oxygen resuscitators commonly use the C size.

C size cylinders have two indexing holes on the cylinder stem, for correct location of the cylinder on to a resuscitator machine. These index holes engage with two protruding pins on the machine's inlet face. There is a seal between the cylinder's outlet hole and the machine's oxygen inlet. This seal is the first location to check if any oxygen leaks are present. Leaks are heard when turning on the oxygen cylinder once the cylinder clamp screw is done up firmly.

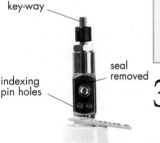

key-way

indexing pin holes

seal removed

3 Before 'cracking' (opening) cylinder, manually remove dust seal completely from full cylinder.

4 To 'crack' a cylinder:
▶ place the oxygen key-wheel on to key-way at end of oxygen cylinder
▶ place one hand halfway down cylinder for stability; with other hand, turn oxygen outlet hole away from yourself and anyone else present—the oxygen jet can cause a nasty friction burn

▷ turn the key-wheel slowly and gently anticlockwise until oxygen flow is heard, then quickly back to the off position, to clear dust or other contaminants from valve area

The new oxygen cylinder is now ready to be connected to equipment.

5 Select appropriate oxygen connecting apparatus.

Assembly of oxygen equipment

To permit the oxygen contained within an oxygen cylinder to be given to a casualty, four basic components are required:
▷ **oxygen cylinder**—preferably full; usually replace for refilling when contents are 1/4 or less
▷ **oxygen regulator** reduces oxygen cylinder pressure
▷ **flow rate control** permits either fixed or variable flow rates of oxygen
▷ **tubing and mask** for effective administration of oxygen to the casualty

Flow meters

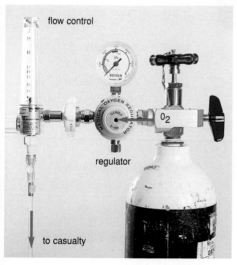

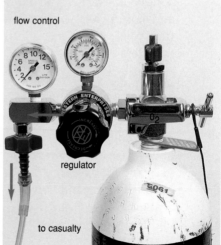

339

Precautions for the Storage and Use of Oxygen

Storage
- medical oxygen is normally stored in black metal cylinders with white shoulders and clearly labelled
- store in a cool, ventilated room which is fire-resistant
- if in the open, protect from dampness and weather
- when almost empty (1/4 or less full), close valve, mark cylinder as 'empty' or 'MT' and store away from full cylinders

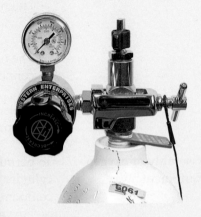

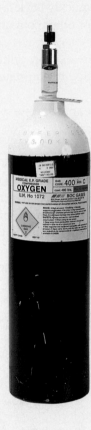

- normally use medical oxygen only—industrial oxygen contains impurities but in an emergency is better than nothing
- **DO NOT** allow petroleum-based grease or oil to come in contact with supply devices on the stem of the cylinder

Care with oxygen
- **DO NOT** drop, drag, roll or slide cylinders (if fractured, the pressure released will turn cylinder into a high-powered missile)
- **DO NOT** use oxygen around an open flame as it will explode
- **DO NOT** allow smoking near oxygen equipment

Rules of use
- only use a cylinder with a proper Australian Standards approved regulating device
- always use correct pressure gauges with oxygen
- ensure 'O' ring and valve seat inserts are clean, dry and in good condition

INFECTION CONTROL AND EQUIPMENT MAINTENANCE

Whenever oxygen equipment has been used:

- precautions must be taken to ensure there is no potential for spread of infection from one casualty to another or to first aider
- prepare it again for immediate use—check regularly; turn cylinder on and off again to check contents

When there is more than one casualty, the first aider should use a new mask for each casualty, making sure that neither the first aider nor the casualties are placed at risk of cross infection.

After use, clean and prepare the equipment for reuse.

- replace disposable parts
- clean and sterilise non-disposable parts

After equipment has been dismantled:

- wipe regulator carefully with damp cloth and antiseptic soap (take care no soap or water enters the unit)
- check that 'O' ring in the handwheel connection is always correctly positioned and in good condition

Those parts of the unit which can be dismantled and need cleaning are cleaned by:

- washing in warm, soapy water
- rinsing in clean, warm water
- rinsing and syringing any airways with clean water
- soaking fittings in an appropriate sterilisation solution
- rinsing fittings in clean, warm water
- allowing fittings to air-dry before reassembling

ADMINISTRATION OF OXYGEN

BREATHING CASUALTY

There is a variety of masks and cannulas available to provide supplementary oxygen to the spontaneously breathing casualty. You should be familiar with their general characteristics. Whatever device is used, it is always important to explain to the casualty what it is and why it is necessary.

Simple universal plastic face mask

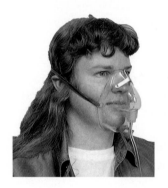

The simple universal plastic face mask can deliver up to 60% oxygen depending on the oxygen flow rate and the casualty's gaseous exchange with each breath. Exhaled air is vented through the holes on each side of the mask. At low oxygen flow rates and deep respirations the casualty may draw in room air through the side holes thereby diluting the oxygen concentrations received. In general a flow rate between 8 and 15 litres per minute (lpm) should ensure adequate oxygen delivery to the casualty. Under a flow rate of 8 lpm with quick respirations, the carbon dioxide doesn't get 'flushed' out of the face mask fully and therefore may have an affect on respirations.

Some casualties tolerate a mask poorly and complain of a feeling of suffocation when the mask is placed over the nose and mouth. Forewarning the casualty that a mask may feel confining but is providing 'more air' than breathing without it may enable the casualty to tolerate the mask with less anxiety. If the casualty cannot tolerate any form of mask over the face then the two-pronged cannula used with oxygen is better than no oxygen at all.

Two-pronged nasal cannula

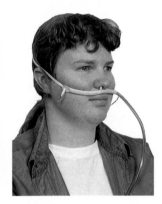

The two-pronged nasal cannula is devised from plastic tubing with two plastic tips that insert into the nostrils. It will deliver oxygen concentration of 30% to 40% with an oxygen flow rate of 3–5 lpm. **Do not use higher flow rates** as they will not increase the delivered oxygen concentration but will cause irritation of the nasal mucosa. The nasal cannula is usually well tolerated but it can cause some soreness around the nostrils and the maximum oxygen concentration it will deliver is limited. This device is the preferred means of oxygen delivery when low to moderate oxygen concentrations are required. It is mainly used for chronic airway disease casualties who are feeling slightly short of breath. Anyone who has acute shortness of breath needs high concentrations of oxygen.

ADMINISTRATION VIA MECHANICAL RESUSCITATOR

There are two major groups of resuscitation systems.

1 **Dependent on a supply of oxygen**
   - oxygen powered: manual or demand valve systems
   - hand powered: softbag and mask systems

2 **Not dependent on a supply of oxygen**
   - aids to expired air resuscitation (e.g. pocket face mask)
   - self-inflating bag and mask systems

Resuscitation systems dependent on a supply of oxygen

Resuscitation systems, whether oxygen powered or hand powered, which depend on a supply of oxygen use one of three types of circuits:

▶ **Non-rebreathing circuits** include a non-return valve which exhausts the expired gas containing carbon dioxide into the atmosphere. High flow rates of oxygen (8–15 lpm) are necessary.

▶ **Partial rebreathing circuits** (semi-closed systems) include a valve system which enables part of the expired gas to be re-inhaled and part to be exhausted to the atmosphere. Carbon dioxide build-up is prevented by a flushing effect, using moderately high flow rates of oxygen (7–10 lpm).

▶ **Rebreathing circuits** (closed circuit systems) include a soda lime absorption system to filter carbon dioxide from the expired gas. The purified gas is then returned to the casualty supplemented with additional oxygen equivalent to that used in the body metabolism. Low flow rates of oxygen (0.5–2 lpm) are used. These units are rarely encountered by first aiders.

Note: Only carbon dioxide is removed, so this system is not suitable for overcoming gas poisoning.

Oxygen powered resuscitators

Demand valve systems

A demand valve oxygen powered resuscitator consists of a non-breathing circuit with a demand valve assembly connected to an oxygen supply.

Breathing Casualty

In breathing casualties inhalation triggers the demand valve and oxygen automatically flows until inhalation is complete. Expired gases pass into the atmosphere.

Non-Breathing Casualty

In non-breathing casualties a manual override is used to inflate the lungs. This is operated by depressing a button directly, or indirectly via a lever. Excess lung pressure is prevented by a pressure relief valve.

TECHNIQUE WITH DEMAND VALVE RESUSCITATORS

Breathing casualty

1 Turn on the oxygen cylinder valve (anticlockwise). Turn on fully and back off 1/4 turn. Check contents gauge for adequate supply.

2 Apply face mask firmly over nose and mouth ensuring an airtight seal. As the casualty breathes in, the resuscitator will automatically supply 100% oxygen until the end of inhalation.

Non-breathing casualty

1 Turn on the oxygen cylinder valve (anticlockwise). Turn on fully and back off 1/4 turn. Check the contents gauge for adequate supply.

2 Position face mask over nose and then mouth area with narrow part of mask between casualty's eyes.

3 Ensure cushion is inflated with normal air pressure. Adjust shape of mask by moulding lead insert.

4 Press down lever on the demand resuscitator until chest commences to rise and then release. Wait until lungs deflate, then repeat operation at the rate of 15 times per minute. The flow rate can be adjusted if a flow control device is fitted. If the chest rises too slowly, move flow rate control device to increase flow rate. If chest rises too quickly, move flow rate control to decrease flow rate. (It is better to have a slower rise rate first and then increase than to have too high a rate which damages the casualty's lungs.)

5 When casualty begins to breathe, stop pressing the lever. The casualty will automatically receive 100% oxygen with each breath on demand.

Hand powered resuscitators

Soft bag and mask systems are preferred by many first aiders as the feel and movements of the bag indicate the condition of the airway, and the presence or absence of breathing. There are two commonly used bag and mask systems which differ basically only in the method of removal of carbon dioxide.

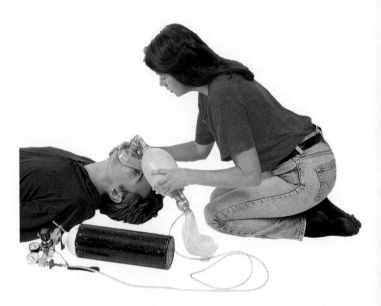

Soft bag and mask partial rebreathing system is commonly used in hospital wards and recovery rooms. High flow rates of oxygen in a partial rebreathing circuit flush out the expired carbon dioxide.

Soft bag and mask closed circuit system operates on rebreathing using low flow rates of oxygen in a closed circuit with soda lime granules to absorb expired carbon dioxide by chemical combination.

Oxygen Administration—General Points

- turn oxygen off after completion of resuscitation

- in suffocation by toxic fumes (e.g. carbon monoxide poisoning) increase flow rate to 8 lpm and leave exhaust valve open to flush system; if casualty not breathing, exhaust valve will need to be intermittently closed for positive pressure ventilation

- if pressure in circuit rises, indicated by over-distension of rebreathing bag, it must be vented by rotating cap of cross valve clockwise to exhaust position, or by lifting mask from casualty's face

- in spontaneously breathing casualties venting of excess gas is automatic if cross valve is turned to intermediate position

- accessories (airways, head harness, therapy equipment and suction tubing) are stored in labelled pockets of the vinyl cover

- oxygen therapy for breathing casualties can be supplied through a fixed restrictor, usually 3 lpm; if required to operate a nebuliser for asthma casualties, a minimum 6 lpm restrictor is necessary to produce an adequate mist

Resuscitation systems not dependent on a supply of oxygen

Self-inflating bag and mask systems
The self-inflating bag and mask systems are identical to the hand powered soft bag and mask systems previously described, except that no oxygen cylinder is connected to the equipment.

USE OF A SOFT BAG RESUSCITATOR ON A NON-BREATHING CASUALTY

1 Kneel at head of casualty.

2 Check, clear and open airway.

3 Insert an oropharyngeal airway (if available).

4 Choose appropriate size face mask (adult or child).

5 Squeeze soft bag to check relief valve and exhalation valve.

6 Place mask over casualty's face (narrow part over bridge of nose).

7 Check mask is firmly applied and that head tilt is maintained.

8 Hold mask with one hand; squeeze bag with other hand and watch for chest to rise; then release bag.

9 Squeeze bag every 4 seconds (adult) or every 3 seconds (child).

10 Check constantly that equipment is functioning and your technique is correct.

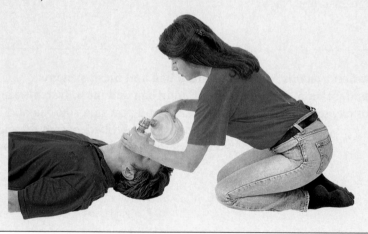

MAINTAINING THE AIRWAY

OROPHARYNGEAL AIRWAY

An oropharyngeal airway is a device used to assist in establishing and maintaining an adequate airway. It may be used in conjunction with a mechanical resuscitator on an unconscious, breathing casualty when difficulty is experienced in maintaining an open airway. It should always be inserted with care.

> **Warning**
>
> - only use on an unconscious casualty (it can irritate the back of throat and cause vomiting, coughing and spasm of larynx)
> - if casualty shows any sign of retching, remove airway device immediately

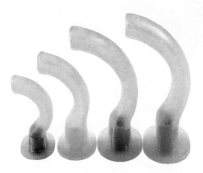

OROPHARYNGEAL ASPIRATION

A sucker is used to aspirate fluid (e.g. mucus, saliva, vomitus fluid) from the mouth and nose to prevent inhalation of the fluid and to obtain and maintain an unobstructed airway. This should only be carried out on an unconscious casualty, otherwise the casualty will gag involuntarily.

Inserting an Oropharyngeal Airway

1 Check casualty's airway is clear.

2 Place oropharyngeal airway on casualty's face to check for correct size—tubing should extend from centre of lips to angle of jaw.

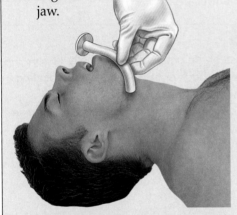

3 To insert, use thumb and index finger crossed to pry the casualty's teeth apart and hold mouth open.

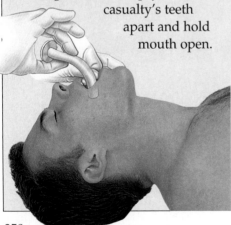

4 Point tip of airway towards roof of casualty's mouth then insert airway approximately 1/3 of its length into casualty's mouth.

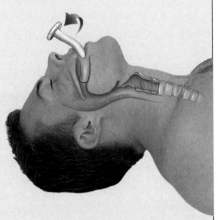

5 Rotate airway over tongue until airway points towards side of casualty's mouth.

6 Gently push airway approximately 2/3 of its length into mouth, rotating so that tip is pointing down the pharynx.

7 Gently push airway further into casualty's mouth until its flange is pressing on lips.

(continued next page)

8   Hyperextend casualty's head and, if necessary, apply a jaw thrust to assist in settling oropharyngeal airway into correct position and maintaining casualty's airway.

Warning: If casualty shows any signs of rejecting the oropharyngeal airway, remove it immediately.

If spinal injury is suspected, care must be taken with any movement of the head.

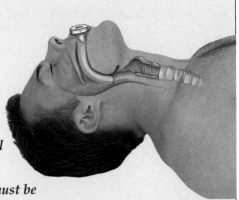

OROPHARYNGEAL ASPIRATION—RIGID SUCTION TUBE (YANKAUER SUCKER)

1   Connect Yankauer sucker to suction tubing.

2   Turn suction source on.

3   Open casualty's mouth with crossed finger technique *(see p. 350)*.

4   Hold suction-head handle by cradling it in curved fingers of one hand, leaving thumb free.

5   Insert suction tube tip into direct-view area of pharynx without open tip of suction-head being blocked (the curve matches mouth and pharynx).

6   Aspirate casualty by blocking hole in tube (adjacent to suction handle) with thumb of hand holding suction-head handle. Aspirate for maximum of 5 seconds.

7   Withdraw suction-head slowly.

8   Ventilate casualty.

9   Before repeating procedure clean equipment by inserting suction-head into a container of water, aspirating water to clear suction-head and tubing.

10   Ensure aspiration bowl does not fill beyond 2/3 full.

Oropharyngeal Aspiration—Flexible Catheter ('Y' Suction Tube)

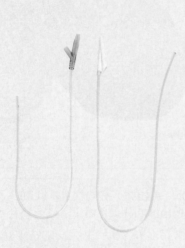

6 Aspirate by blocking Y piece on catheter with a finger and rotating catheter continuously during removal—aspirate for a maximum of 5 seconds at any one time.

7 Allow casualty to breathe oxygen, or ventilate casualty.

8 Before repeating procedure, insert catheter into a container of water, aspirating the water to clear catheter and tubing.

1 Connect appropriate size Y suction catheter to end of suction tubing.

9 Ensure aspiration bowl does not fill beyond 2/3 full.

2 Turn suction source on.

10 If an oropharyngeal airway is in place, carry out above procedure, aspirating either side of oropharyngeal air way as well as the inside.

3 Determine maximum length of catheter by measuring dis tance from corner of casualty's nose to the earlobe (place catheter against face).

Note: DO NOT leave suction turned on unnecessarily as it wastes oxygen at approximately 20 lpm.

4 Open casualty's mouth with crossed fingers technique *(see p. 350).*

5 Insert catheter to appropriate depth with Y piece open.

ASSESSING RESPIRATORY EFFORT

Oxygen therapy must be administered at an appropriate flow rate for the wellbeing of the casualty. To ensure this, it is important to continue to monitor the casualty throughout the procedure.

Oxygen is given to an adult once every 4 seconds (15 times per minute) and to a child every 3 seconds (20 times per minute). Pulse and breathing should then be checked for up to 10 seconds before ventilation is continued at the same rate. The first aider should continue to monitor the pulse and breathing about every minute until medical aid arrives.

In giving oxygen, it is important to ensure the chest rises slowly (the slower the better) because long, very slow inhalations are more effective.

For the non-breathing casualty, the oxygen flow rate is set so that the amount of oxygen administered is just sufficient to inflate the lungs. This is to prevent any excess oxygen going into the stomach where it could possibly cause distension and regurgitation.

Defibrillation

Defibrillation is the giving of a controlled electric shock to the heart to restore its normal rhythm. This is necessary when the electrical impulses of the heart become chaotic so that the heart muscle no longer contracts effectively and rhythmically. This condition is called ventricular fibrillation. It may cause the heart to stop completely (cardiac arrest).

The first aider cannot distinguish between fibrillation and cardiac arrest as the pulse is not detectable in either case. Defibrillation equipment assesses the heart's activity and ascertains whether defibrillation should be applied. Not all abnormal rhythms after cardiac arrests are reversible. If the heart does not have any electrical activity there is no benefit in giving defibrillation. Defibrillators are not to be used on a person under 12 years old.

EFFECTS OF DEFIBRILLATION

If cardiac arrest occurs after a heart attack, defibrillation is the procedure most likely to promote recovery of normal rhythm. Defibrillation is most effective when carried out within 3 minutes of a cardiac arrest, its effectiveness decreasing with time. Good CPR helps to prolong the time during which effective defibrillation can be achieved.

Although some casualties have made good recoveries after being 'arrested' for longer periods, it is vital to get a defibrillator as soon as possible to a casualty who is not breathing and has no pulse.

There are two main groups of cardiac arrest casualties:

► those in whom a cardiac event is the cause of cardiac arrest

► those whose cardiac arrest is secondary to non-cardiac causes (e.g. drowning or blood loss from trauma)

Casualties in the first of these groups are usually conscious until cardiac arrest occurs and are more likely to have the arrest reversed. Casualties in the second group can be effectively treated only if the underlying cause is dealt with.

USE OF DEFIBRILLATION EQUIPMENT

The semi-automatic external defibrillator (SAED) has been shown to be safe and effective in the hands of trained first aiders. *SAEDs must only be used by authorised personnel*. Adhesive defibrillator pads are attached to the casualty in the usual pad positions *(see p. 357)*. The pulse is checked and if none present, the 'Analyse' key is pressed by the operator or the machine will analyse automatically—depending on make/model of defibrillator. The SAED makes a diagnosis of the heart rhythm. It then advises the operator whether to shock the casualty or not, by displaying messages on a screen and/or by voice prompts.

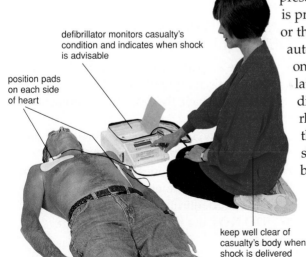

defibrillator monitors casualty's condition and indicates when shock is advisable

position pads on each side of heart

keep well clear of casualty's body when shock is delivered

To deliver a shock, the operator must press the 'Shock' key which is only active if a shockable rhythm is diagnosed. The SAED will then advise everyone to stand clear and will then deliver the shock.

Casualties with permanent pacemakers can be safely defibrillated (check for a minor scar near left collarbone—above heart). The pacemaker will most likely have failed, or you would not need to defibrillate. Proceed as with any other casualty.

Before taking a defibrillator for use in the field, make sure you have:

- 1 spare battery
- 1 automatic module (if applicable)
- 1 rough face washer (to wipe casualty's chest)
- 1 paper towel
- 1 shaver
- 1 pair scissors (to cut clothing)
- disposable gloves
- 2 defibrillator pads (store in a cool environment and keep flat)

CARE IN THE USE OF DEFIBRILLATORS

- ensure all personnel are clear of the casualty before discharging the shock
- **DO NOT** have the casualty in contact with metal fixtures
- ensure oxygen equipment is switched off during defibrillation
- ensure mobile phones and radios are switched off, or at least 6 metres away
- **NEVER** defibrillate in a moving vehicle
- **DO NOT** use in a wet environment

> regular checks should be made of defibrillation equipment
> **DO NOT** fold self-adhesive pads
> regularly have the equipment serviced by authorised agents

MANAGEMENT OF DEFIBRILLATION
(requires two first aiders—one trained and authorised to use SAEDs)

1 Follow DRABC. **DRABC**

2 Establish casualty is unconscious, has no pulse and is not breathing.

3 Commence CPR, and continue during following steps.

4 Expose casualty's chest.

5 Remove patches, jewellery etc.

6 Check for pacemaker.

7 Wipe chest to ensure it is dry—shave chest if hairy.

8 Attach cables to defibrillator pads.

9 Attach pads to casualty's chest:
  • one electrode cable and pad to casualty's right chest wall (below collarbone)
  • one electrode cable and pad to casualty's left side chest wall (below left nipple).

10 Stop CPR.

11 Ensure everyone is clear of casualty.

12 Press 'On' switch firmly.

13 Press 'Analyse' button or machine will analyse automatically—depending on make/model of defibrillator.

14 Follow machine's instructions.

DEFIBRILLATION WITH CHILDREN

In children, non-cardiac causes of cardiac arrest such as drowning or suffocation predominate. In such cases there is unlikely to be heart electrical activity, and defibrillation is therefore unlikely to be of assistance.

Remember: DO NOT defibrillate anyone under 12 years old.

Chapter

21

Cardiovascular emergencies

Cardiovascular disease is the big killer in Australia. Of those who die from a cardio-vascular disease, heart disease claims the greatest number.

Chest pain or discomfort is an important symptom. However, not all chest pain and discomfort are caused by cardiovascular disease. Some chest pain may result from less serious conditions. Conversely, not all heart emergencies are accompanied by chest pain or discomfort.

This chapter discusses how to deal with chest pain and discomfort, what each cardiovascular disease is and how to recognise and manage it. Importantly, this chapter will explain when it is necessary to seek medical help urgently.

CARDIOVASCULAR EMERGENCIES

Cardiovascular disease (diseases of the heart and circulatory system) can develop from an early age. Inappropriate diet and lack of exercise are considered contributing factors.

Although the proportion of people who die each year from cardiovascular disease has been declining since the 1960s, it is still the number one cause of death in Australia.

Who will develop cardiovascular disease?

Some people are more at risk than others. Men are more likely to develop heart disease than women—although the difference decreases with increasing age. Also at higher risk are people of lower socio-economic status, those who have a family history of heart disease, and indigenous Australians. Other factors which increase the risk of cardiovascular disease include:

- smoking
- a diet high in fats
- high blood pressure (hypertension)
- high blood cholesterol levels
- obesity
- lack of regular exercise
- diabetes

When people suffer from a combination of risk factors—such as smoking and high blood pressure—the possibility of a heart attack or stroke is substantially increased.

CARDIOVASCULAR DISORDERS

High blood pressure and atherosclerosis (narrowing of the arteries) can be the first indicators of cardiovascular disease. They can lead to cardiovascular emergencies such as heart attack, angina, stroke, and cardiac arrest.

High blood pressure (hypertension)

Blood pressure—the pressure of blood against the inside walls of the arteries—will quite normally go up and down depending on such factors as the level of excitement or emotional stress.

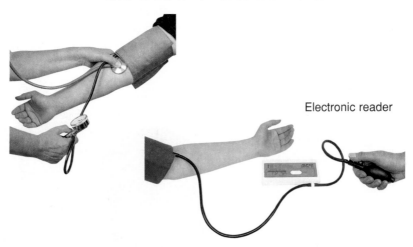

Electronic reader

In most people, blood pressure will come down when the excitement or stress is over. In some people, especially those with a family history of high blood pressure, the blood pressure remains high all the time. This is termed hypertension. Over time, hypertension damages the tissues of the cardiovascular system, increasing risk of heart attack, heart failure, stroke, and eye and kidney problems.

Atherosclerosis (narrowing of the arteries)

Narrowing of the arteries occurs when fatty deposits (cholesterol) build up on the inner walls of arteries. This may remain undetected for years. In the coronary arteries it is called coronary artery disease.

As an artery gets narrower, less and less blood can get through. Atherosclerosis often begins in childhood although symptoms may not be obvious until middle age or later. Some studies have shown that coronary artery disease begins in teenage years, perhaps due to a high fat diet, and is worse in smokers.

Signs and symptoms of atherosclerosis begin when a narrowed section of artery prevents the tissues beyond from getting enough oxygenated blood for normal functioning.

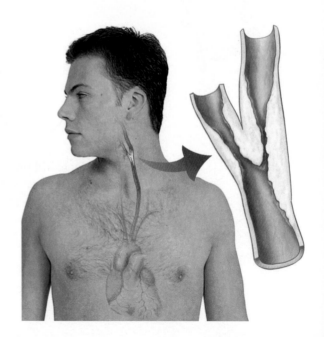

CHEST PAIN OR DISCOMFORT

> **Warning**
>
> Any unusual chest pain or discomfort should be taken seriously.

Although chest pain unrelated to injury can be caused by stress, indigestion, disorders of the oesophagus, and muscle spasm, it can also be the result of cardiovascular disease and a sign of a heart attack or angina. The first aider does not have medical expertise in diagnosis and should assume a 'worst-case' scenario.

Pain may feel like:

heaviness

tightness

squeezing

pressure

crushing

vice-like

indigestion

aching jaw

sore arm

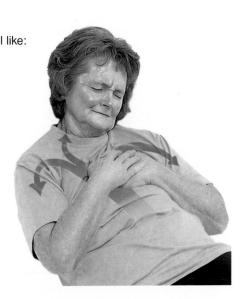

If the pain is heart-related, it indicates that the amount of blood flowing through the coronary arteries is not sufficient for the heart's needs.

MANAGEMENT OF CHEST PAIN OR DISCOMFORT

Anyone who suffers chest pain or discomfort should see a doctor. The only time medical aid is not necessary is when a person known to have angina gets pain relief quickly after taking the prescribed medication.

1 Importance of rest
- treat situation as life-threatening even if casualty denies seriousness of symptoms
- advise casualty to stop what they are doing, and sit or lie down and rest
- sitting upright can often be the most comfortable position for those experiencing chest pain.

2 Medication
- if casualty has a history of heart disease and has medication for pain, help by getting the medication (do not give more than usual dose)
- nitrates (e.g. glyceryl trinitrate and isosorbide dinitrate) are used to control angina and are most commonly taken in a tablet held under tongue or as an aerosol spray.

3 Urgent medical attention
When chest pain or discomfort is associated with cardio-vascular disease, survival often depends on early medical care:
- ☎ *call 000 for an ambulance immediately*
- **DO NOT** drive the casualty to hospital as cardiac arrest can happen at any time
- give a conscious casualty 300 mg (one tablet) of aspirin in water, unless casualty is allergic to aspirin, is an asthmatic or is already taking anti-coagulant med-ication (e.g. warfarin).

Note: Aspirin is taken to minimise chances of more blood clots forming not to reduce chest pain or discomfort.

4 Monitoring vital signs
- while waiting for ambulance, calm the casualty, and monitor vital signs
- be prepared to give CPR.

ANGINA

Chest pain or discomfort may be brought on by emotional stress or exercise, because narrowed coronary arteries are unable to supply the additional blood needed when the heart's activity increases.

Signs and symptoms

Relative lack of blood supply, with a consequent build up of waste products, causes pain or discomfort in the chest which may spread to the neck, jaw, shoulders and arms. This type of chest pain is usually identified by a feeling of pressure, burning or tightness in the centre of the chest. It is known as angina (angina pectoris) and can usually be relieved by rest, and/or prescribed medication.

MANAGEMENT OF ANGINA

1 Support casualty in sitting position.

2 Encourage rest and provide reassurance.

3 Loosen tight clothing around neck, chest and waist.

4 Tell casualty to either place prescribed dose of angina tablets under tongue or inside cheek as per directions on bottle,

OR
administer Nitro-Lingual spray under the tongue.

5 If pain and discomfort persist for longer than 10 minutes after rest, ☎ *Call 000 for an ambulance immediately.*

6 Give the conscious casualty 300mg (one tablet) of aspirin in water, unless casualty is allergic to aspirin, is an asthmatic or is already taking anti-coagulant medication (e.g. warfarin)

HEART ATTACK

A heart attack occurs when part of the heart muscle is damaged because its supply of oxygenated blood has been cut off. The usual cause is a blood clot stuck in a coronary artery narrowed by atherosclerosis. If the blood supply is not restored within an hour, part of the damaged heart muscle begins to die.

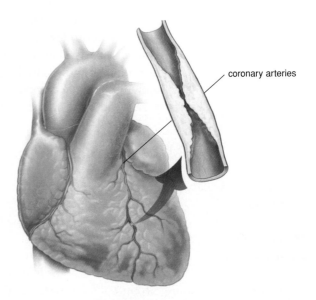

coronary arteries

Damaged heart muscle may initiate an uncontrolled disorganised rhythm (ventricular fibrillation) which may cause the heart to stop beating. This is cardiac arrest.

If the casualty has a form of chest pain or discomfort similar to angina but which is not relieved by medication and rest, the first aider should manage it as a heart attack.

Signs and symptoms

Pain or discomfort associated with a heart attack is persistent and usually gives a crushing sense of pressure or burning in the centre of the chest. This may be accompanied by sweating, shortness of breath and a sick feeling. The pain may spread in all directions—to the back, neck and arms. Half of those who die from cardiac arrest do so in the first 3–4 hours, so it is important to act quickly.

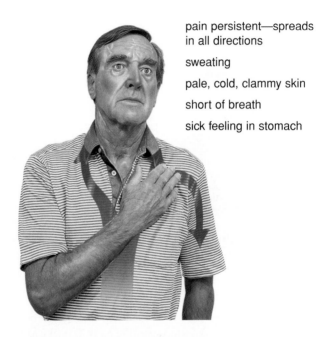

pain persistent—spreads in all directions

sweating

pale, cold, clammy skin

short of breath

sick feeling in stomach

Many people experiencing a heart attack delay seeking care. They do not realise they are having a heart attack or simply associate the symptoms with indigestion or muscle soreness. The symptoms of heart attack may seem, to the casualty, to be simply a sensation of discomfort. To delay treatment is to risk sudden death through cardiac arrest.

MANAGEMENT OF HEART ATTACK

1 Follow DRABC.

2 **If casualty conscious**: place in sitting position.

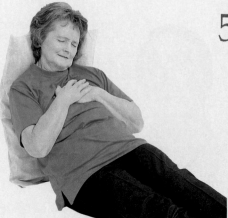

If casualty unconscious: turn on side in recovery position.

3 ☎ *Call 000 for an ambulance immediately.*

4 Loosen tight clothing.

5 Give the conscious casualty 300 mg (one tablet) of aspirin in water, unless the casualty is allergic to aspirin, is an asthmatic or is already taking anti-coagulant medication (e.g. warfarin).

MANAGEMENT OF CARDIAC ARREST

1 Follow DRABC.

2 ☎ *Call 000 for an ambulance immediately.*

CONGESTIVE HEART FAILURE

Congestive heart failure is a condition in which the heart cannot pump normally. It usually develops as a result of old age or chronic heart disease.

Signs and symptoms

▶ a general feeling of tiredness
▶ breathlessness when exercising
▶ swollen feet, ankles, legs and abdomen
▶ coughing and wheezing

With advanced congestive heart failure, the casualty may feel breathless even when resting and may have to sit up to be comfortable.

MANAGEMENT OF CONGESTIVE HEART FAILURE

1 Follow DRABC. **DRABC**

2 ☎ *Call 000 for an ambulance immediately.*

3 If casualty conscious, place in sitting position.

4 Reassure casualty and loosen tight clothing.

STROKE

Unlike other cardiovascular emergencies, a stroke does not cause chest pain. A stroke occurs when an artery taking blood to the brain becomes blocked or bursts. In most cases, this is the result of a clot at a part of an artery narrowed by long-term build-up of fatty deposits. As a result of a stroke, brain cells may be damaged and functions controlled by that part of the brain affected.

Paralysis of parts of the body or speech problems are common after a stroke. Although many people make a good recovery, a stroke can be fatal.

Sometimes the person will get warnings of a future stroke. These 'mini strokes' have the same symptoms as a stroke but are temporary and do not cause long-term harm to the brain. They are caused by temporary disruptions to the brain's blood supply. **Seek medical attention as a future stroke may be preventable.**

People most at risk of a stroke are those who are elderly, have high blood pressure, smoke, have heart disease or diabetes, or have previously had a stroke.

A stroke is a life-threatening emergency.

Signs and symptoms

▸ weakness or paralysis, especially on one side of body

▸ feeling of numbness in face, arm or leg

▸ difficulty speaking or understanding

▸ unexplained dizziness

▸ disturbed vision

▸ loss of balance

▸ confusion

Inability to communicate when otherwise alert can cause extreme anxiety in the casualty. Grasp both hands and ask the casualty to squeeze. Usually casualty will respond with one or other hand. Then communicate by hand squeezes—one for yes and two for no. Be calm and reassuring.

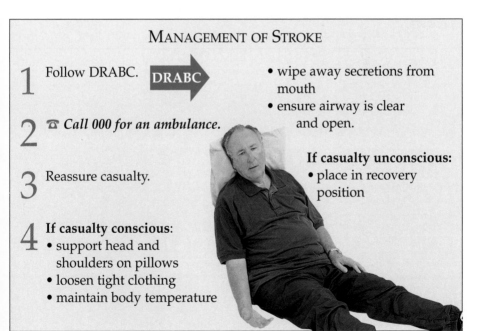

MANAGEMENT OF STROKE

1 Follow DRABC. **DRABC**

2 ☎ *Call 000 for an ambulance.*

3 Reassure casualty.

4 **If casualty conscious:**
  • support head and shoulders on pillows
  • loosen tight clothing
  • maintain body temperature

• wipe away secretions from mouth
• ensure airway is clear and open.

If casualty unconscious:
• place in recovery position

MANAGEMENT OF CARDIOVASCULAR EMERGENCIES

Angina	Heart attack	Cardiac arrest	Congestive heart failure	Stroke
sitting position	DRABC	DRABC	DRABC	DRABC
rest		☎ *Call 000*	☎ *Call 000*	☎ *Call 000*
loosen tight clothing	sitting position, if conscious			
casualty take medication	☎ *Call 000*		sitting position, if conscious	loosen tight clothing
seek medical aid if pain persists	loosen clothing		loosen clothing	ensure airway clear

Childbirth

Most expectant parents will have attended classes to prepare themselves for the birth of their baby. Nevertheless, all parents expecting their first child, or mothers-to-be who have gone into labour unexpectedly need special support.

Reassuring the woman and remaining calm will help her to stay calm. This will help her to remember the procedures she has been taught and to deal with the labour more comfortably.

Labour usually lasts for several hours and in most cases proceeds normally. There is generally plenty of time to arrange for transport to hospital or to seek medical assistance.

This chapter outlines the procedures for delivering a baby safely, even when the birth is not entirely straightforward.

CHILDBIRTH PREPARATION

Childbirth is a natural process and the majority of babies are born without complications during delivery. First aid assistance may be necessary if the baby starts to come before its due time, if the woman lives in a remote part of the country or if an emergency occurs which threatens the life of the mother or the baby. In any of these situations, assistance with the delivery of the baby and care for the mother may be necessary, until an ambulance, midwife or medical practitioner arrives.

Note: If you encounter a birth away from medical assistance or access to an ambulance service, call for urgent medical advice, using a telephone, mobile phone, or Royal Flying Doctor Service radio for continuing advice during delivery.

INFECTION

Infection is a serious danger to both mother and baby. It is essential to minimise the risk of infection.

- ▶ wash your hands, nails and forearms thoroughly with warm water and soap (if possible)
- ▶ wear disposable gloves if available

PREPARING FOR THE BIRTH

Childbirth is a very personal and emotional time for the parents, and may also be for the first aider. Preparation is essential, as well as calmness and reassurance.

The expectant mother will experience pain and strong emotions, and will have to work hard to deliver the baby. She may feel afraid, not know what to expect and want the support of someone close to her (such as the baby's father or a female friend). There will be blood and probably noise during the birth and the woman will need assistance to maintain her breathing pattern to aid the birth.

For the birth, the expectant mother can be on any flat surface, although if she finds this uncomfortable, she may wish to squat or adopt some other comfortable position. If in a public area, ask others to move away to give the mother privacy. As a first aider, you can:

▶ prepare a suitable clean surface for the mother
  • a large plastic sheet to go under her
  • a clean sheet to place over the plastic
▶ boil water to sterilise scissors for cutting the cord.
▶ collect other materials needed

FIRST AIDER'S CHILDBIRTH KIT

- 1 large plastic sheet
- 2 clean cotton sheets
- 3 bunny rugs
- towels
- large plastic bags for soiled linen
- 3 sterile or clean cord ties (e.g. string, linen tape) each about 8 cm long

- sterile scissors
- gauze swabs or a clean soft cloth
- sanitary pads/disposable nappies
- disposable gloves
- large plastic bag for placenta

THE BIRTH

FIRST STAGE—ONSET OF LABOUR

The first stage of labour usually lasts less than 12 hours. However, a woman who has already had a child may progress through this stage very rapidly. Early contractions may begin as an aching feeling in the lower abdomen.

Signs—first stage

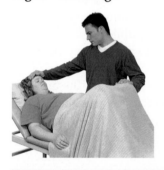

Signs usually include one or all of the following:
- ▶ cramp-like pains in lower abdomen every 2–15 minutes, each lasting 30–60 seconds increasing in frequency and duration
- ▶ a 'show' of bloodstained mucus—the plug which sealed the cervix during pregnancy
- ▶ the 'waters breaking'—a sudden rush, or sometimes a constant trickle, of amniotic fluid indicates the sac containing the baby has broken—note the colour and consistency and inform medical aid.

MANAGEMENT OF FIRST STAGE

Management of first stage

1 Reassure the woman.

2 Keep her comfortable.

3 ☎ *Call 000 for an ambulance.*

4 If the ambulance will be delayed, begin to collect the materials needed.

Preparation for second stage

1 Assist the woman into a comfortable position. If the woman is most comfortable on her back, then ensure her upper body is raised.

2 Help in removing any clothing that may be in the way during delivery. Warm baby blankets (bunny rugs).

Note: As the first stage may take a number of hours, the woman may wish to move around.

SECOND STAGE—THE BIRTH

The second stage begins when the cervix (neck of the womb) is fully dilated (widened) and ends with the birth of the baby.

There are a number of potential dangers for the mother and baby during the birth.

▶ mother
  • infection
  • bleeding

▶ baby
  • infection from the cut end of umbilical cord
  • cold
  • lack of oxygen

Signs—second stage

Contractions may alter in frequency and duration. They will be quite intense at this stage and the woman will feel the urge to 'bear down'. As the cervix may not be fully dilated at this stage, discourage the woman from pushing. Ask her to open her mouth and pant during each contraction until help arrives as the baby is usually safer inside than out. The woman may push anyway either voluntary or involuntary.

Most babies are born head first. As the baby is about to be born, the top of the head can be seen at the opening to the birth canal. This is called 'crowning'. There will be an increased flow of bloodstained mucus and the mother may feel the need to have a bowel movement. **DO NOT let her sit on the toilet.**

MANAGEMENT OF SECOND STAGE

First aider's preparations

1 Tie apron or sheet around waist to protect clothing and minimise infection.

2 Wash and dry hands thoroughly and put on disposable gloves if available.

3 Prepare two warmed blankets, towels or nappies for the baby.

Prepare woman for delivery

1 Wash the area from the entrance to the vagina to the anus using soap and water and a clean swab for each stroke (wipe from front to back).

2 When head is crowning, encourage the mother to:
- stop pushing
- keep her mouth open and pant (fast, shallow breaths), as the baby's head is delivering
- rest between contractions.

Normal delivery with head presenting first

1 Control baby's head with gentle but steady pressure from the direction of the mother's pubic area down-wards—the head will usually appear with the face towards the mother's anus but will then rotate to face one side.

2 Check whether umbilical cord is around the baby's neck:
- if cord is around the neck, free it by easing it carefully over the baby's head if at all possible (but do not pull on it)
- if this is not possible, tie the cord in two places using sterile string (or bootlaces) and then cut between the two ties (use sterile scissors).

3 Support the baby's head in palms of your hands and wait.

4 During the next contraction, the baby's shoulders will be delivered:
- hold baby under the armpits
- lift baby up towards the mother's stomach.

5 Note the time baby was born.

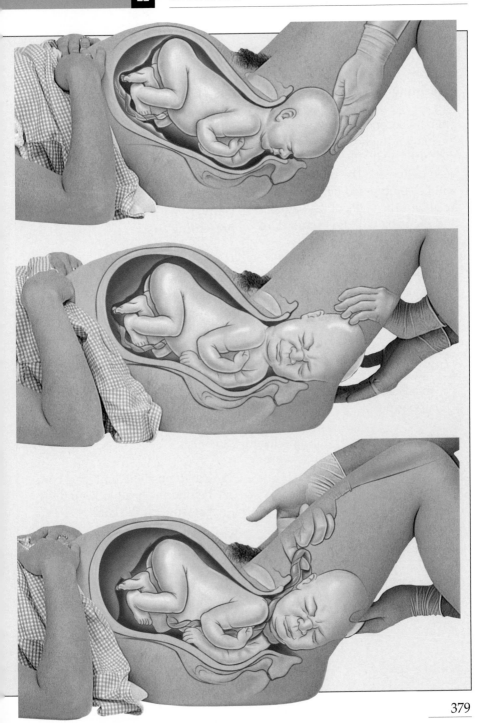

MANAGEMENT OF SECOND STAGE—COMPLICATIONS

Delivery with buttocks or foot presenting first (breech birth)

This can become life-threatening for the baby if the head gets stuck in the birth canal after the body has been delivered. The umbilical cord will be compressed between the head and the walls of the vagina, and the baby will die from lack of oxygen.

1 Place mother in a position (for example on the very edge of bed) that allows the baby to be delivered downwards.

2 Allow mother to push the baby out herself—gently guide baby to ensure the back remains uppermost.

3 After delivery of hips and legs, wrap body of baby in a warm blanket.

4 After delivery of shoulders allow the baby to 'hang' downwards.

5 When the nape of the neck is visible:
  • lift the baby's body upwards by the ankles, while supporting the body.
  • allow the head to deliver slowly.

Delivery with umbilical cord presenting first

This is a life-threatening situation because the cord will be compressed and the flow of oxygenated blood to the baby stopped. The baby could die within minutes.

1 Place mother in a kneeling position with head down and buttocks right up in the air.

2 Seek urgent medical advice.

3 Try to push the umbilical cord behind the head to keep the pressure off the cord.

Note: Inform mother of seriousness of this situation.

IMMEDIATE CARE OF THE BABY

Immediately after birth, the baby will be wet and slippery. Take care not to drop the baby or pull on the cord. The baby may be blue at birth and must be kept warm. Leave the umbilical cord intact and, supporting the baby's head, neck and shoulders with one hand, and feet with the other:

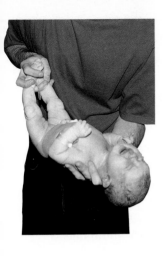

- place baby's head low to drain secretions from mouth and nose
- dry baby quickly and thoroughly with a fresh, clean towel
- place baby on mother's stomach—(if no resuscitation necessary) and encourage baby to breast-feed, this aids with keeping baby warm and maternal bonding
- wrap baby in warmed towel or blanket to keep it warm

Most babies will cry straightaway, an indication of breathing. As they start breathing, they change from blue to pink (the hands and feet may remain blue for several hours).

If the baby does not breathe straightaway, try stimulating it by gently rubbing its back. **DO NOT** hold the baby upside down by the heels and slap it on the back or the buttocks to make it cry.

If the baby does not cry or show signs of breathing after 1 minute, clear the airway of mucus with your fingers and perform EAR. To perform EAR on a baby, seal your mouth over the mouth and nose together. Blow gently—just enough to see the chest rise. Do this 30 times per minute.

In such cases inflation is nearly always the primary need of the newborn, not chest compression. Chest compressions on a newborn should **NOT** be attempted by persons untrained in neonatal resuscitation. The pulse is difficult to measure in the newborn but may be detectable by lightly holding the base of the umbilical cord between the thumb and index finger.

MANAGEMENT OF THE THIRD STAGE—THE AFTERBIRTH

The afterbirth (placenta) is normally not delivered until 10 minutes or more after the birth of the baby. It is expelled by contractions of the uterus. To help delivery of afterbirth:

1   Help mother into a comfortable position, as for the birth.

2   If cord is long enough, encourage mother to put baby to her breast (this will help uterus to contract, expelling afterbirth and controlling bleeding)—**DO NOT PULL ON CORD** as this may cause excessive bleeding.

3   Retain afterbirth in a plastic bag for medical inspection.

4   Give mother hot or cold drinks and offer a light snack (provided afterbirth has been delivered).

After **delivery of afterbirth**, the mother may continue to bleed. Normally, there is enough blood to fill a sanitary pad every 5 minutes.

If there is a great deal of blood or the flow is not slowing down or it increases suddenly:

1   ☎ *Call 000 for an ambulance* (if not already summoned).

2   Massage the mother's lower abdomen until it becomes firm (this will help reduce excessive bleeding).

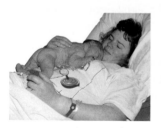

CARE OF THE MOTHER

Once the mother has given birth, she will feel exhausted and may have 'the shakes'. Depending on circumstances and her wishes, the following will help her regain strength and minimise risk of infection:

▶   clean birth canal area with clean towels or gauze pads

▶   sponge her face, hands and legs and help her to change any soiled clothing

▶   place a sanitary pad or disposable nappy in position

▶   give her hot or cold drinks and offer a light snack (provided afterbirth has been delivered)

Care of the umbilical cord
Once the baby is pink and breathing, it does not need the blood supply from umbilical cord. After delivery of afterbirth, tie the cord **only** if there is a long delay expected before the arrival of the ambulance.

If the cord has to be tied:

1 Firmly tie with sterile string (bootlaces etc.) in 3 places— 10 cm, 15 cm and 20 cm from the baby's navel (cord must be tied securely to prevent bleeding after it is cut).

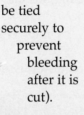

As cutting the cord increases risk of bleeding and infection, it is necessary only if:
- there are complications during delivery (see p. 380)
- baby needs to be resuscitated and must be moved away from the mother
- mother needs attention and cannot hold baby
- cord is too short for mother to hold baby properly
- birth is in a remote area which is isolated from medical aid

If the cord has to be cut:

1 Cut between the 2nd and 3rd tie away from the baby.

2 Cover stump of cord loosely with a sterile dressing.

3 Check cord for bleeding every 15 minutes for first hour then half hourly until medical aid arrives.

▷ cover her with a warm blanket
▷ check her pulse, temperature and respiration
▷ check blood loss regularly—gently massage lower abdomen to control excessive bleeding
▷ encourage her to rest while waiting for medical aid

Once mother and baby have been cared for:
▷ retain all bloodstained material in plastic bags for medical inspection (separate bags for used sanitary pads)
▷ clean all surfaces contaminated by blood and body fluids

Vaginal Bleeding and Miscarriage

Miscarriage is the loss of the foetus before the twentieth week of pregnancy. This usually occurs because the foetus was not developing properly and was not able to survive.

A woman who miscarries is in danger of going into shock. She may be frightened and very distressed and reluctant to accept the help of a male first aider.

Signs and symptoms

▶ vaginal bleeding (this may be severe)
▶ signs of shock
▶ cramp-like pains in lower abdomen
▶ aching in lower back
▶ expelling of foetus or tissue

Management of Miscarriage

1 ☎ *Call 000 for an ambulance.*

2 Help woman into a comfortable position.

3 Have her place towel or sanitary pad over her vulva.

4 Monitor bleeding (do not try to control) and pulse—record details every 10 minutes.

5 Help to maintain normal body temperature.

6 Keep any expelled material and give to medical personnel.

7 Do not give anything to eat or drink as she may need an operation.

23

Emotionally disturbed casualties

First aiders sometimes need to care for casualties who are emotionally disturbed. The disturbance may be due to a number of factors, or a combination of any of these: the casualty's mental health or general state of mind, the effect of drugs or alcohol, reactions following an accident or trauma. Even aggressive or violent behaviour could be the result of deeply distressing and fearful emotions, so the first aider needs to be able to respond appropriately.

The emotionally disturbed casualty is often someone you know. It is less common to have to deal with an emotionally disturbed person who is a complete stranger.

First aiders must aim to cope with the situation while at the same time protecting the casualty, themselves and anyone else at the scene, until professional help arrives. Communication skills, especially listening, are your greatest asset. Body language, both the first aider's and the casualty's, can also be very important.

This chapter looks at the more common types of emotional disturbance and ways of dealing with them.

Psychological Trauma

Psychological trauma is experienced when a person is faced with a threat to life. Trauma is also likely to be experienced when one's child or close family member is threatened. Trauma is especially likely if the threat is unexpected, apparently inescapable, and beyond usual experience. Psychological trauma often accompanies physical injury, particularly when the injury is the result of accidents, criminal assault, natural disasters, war, or community violence. It may therefore accompany some of the situations which involve the first aider in managing physical injuries.

Children experience an acute stress reaction similar to that of adults. However, the severity of their signs and symptoms is closely related to whether or not they are separated from their families. Their recovery is closely connected to the recovery of those who care for them.

ACUTE STRESS REACTION

Almost everyone exposed to psychological trauma will have an acute stress reaction. Casualties are more likely to recover from an acute stress reaction if the first aider is calm, competent, and compassionate.

Signs and symptoms

The signs and symptoms of acute stress reaction are caused by the flooding of the mind with stress and by attempts to block stress out of the mind. Children have similar reactions to adults, but they may have more difficulty expressing feelings in words. Signs and symptoms include:

> tension, trembling, nausea, insomnia, nightmares

> fear, sadness, bitterness, irritability, anger, blaming other people, rapid mood changes

> confusion, forgetfulness, inability to concentrate

> images of the experience intruding into the mind, feeling as though the experience is happening all over again

> shock, disbelief, numbness, feeling as though what happened is unreal

> wanting to be alone, feeling that nobody could understand what they have been through, feeling guilty about being a survivor

MANAGEMENT OF ACUTE STRESS REACTION

The first aider can help with practical needs and by caring, listening, and giving information.

1 Help casualty reunite with family members or friends.

2 Help casualty tell you what is needed. If this is not possible, anticipate needs (e.g. drink, warmth, food, family).

3 Be a good listener. Encourage casualty to tell what happened and express feelings. Don't interrupt. Don't reassure falsely. Don't try to talk casualty out of these feelings or say that others are worse off.

4 Don't take it personally if the casualty is angry or blames others. Stay calm, involved and understanding.

5 After casualty has told what happened, reassure that these feelings are to be expected after trauma.

6 If the casualty can't talk about what happened or express feelings, sit quietly and give support by your presence.

POST-TRAUMATIC STRESS DISORDER

In some cases, after several weeks of acute stress reaction, the casualty develops a more long-lasting problem—post-traumatic stress disorder.

Signs and symptoms

▷ repeated nightmares, flashbacks and images of the trauma

▷ emotional numbness, loss of memory of the experience

▷ fear and avoidance of reminders of the trauma

▷ physical reactions to reminders of the trauma (e.g. racing heart, rapid breathing, sweating)

By offering calm, compassionate support soon after trauma, the first aider can help prevent post-traumatic stress disorder.

GRIEF

Grief is a normal process enabling a person to gradually come to terms with the loss of a loved one. Grief can also follow serious physical injury (e.g. after accidents). People grieve in different ways. Loss has a greater impact if it is unexpected, sudden, or involves a child. The initial grief response is often of shock or disbelief. Over subsequent weeks and months, the grieving person experiences waves of sadness, heartache, and mental images of the lost person. Insomnia, loss of appetite, loss of interest, and poor concentration are usual.

MANAGEMENT OF GRIEF

1 Reunite casualty with surviving family members, if possible.

2 Provide space, privacy, and emotional support.

3 Encourage casualty to express feelings. Accept the feelings. Don't try to reassure casualty or cheer them up.

Psychiatric Casualties

Always treat people with a psychiatric illness with the same politeness and respect with which you treat others. Although a casualty may appear thought-disordered or violent, for example, the majority will remember the details of the situation—often with extreme embarrassment or shame—and the treatment given. Wherever possible reassure accompanying family, friends, and onlookers, who may be confused or deeply upset.

General Management

Protect yourself and others from getting hurt. Don't get closely involved unless you are convinced it is safe.

1 **If you judge it is not safe:**
☎ *call 000 for emergency services.*

If you judge it is safe:
• approach the casualty, and identify yourself as a first aider.

2 Check vital signs, if casualty gives you permission to do so.

3 Check casualty's level of consciousness by asking name, address, date, and whereabouts.

4 Stay calm, positive, and open. Be polite and respectful.

5 Encourage casualty to tell you what is on their mind. Listen closely.

6 Don't interrupt, contradict, argue, or falsely reassure casualty. Don't scold, slap, or attempt to restrain casualty.

7 ☎ *Call 000 for emergency services* when you have enough information.

PANIC

Signs and symptoms

▶ anxiety, fear, terror, and a feeling of impending disaster

▶ racing heart, cold sweaty palms, rapid breathing, enlarged pupils, tremor

▶ headache, lump in the throat, breathlessness, a feeling of constriction or pain in the chest, diarrhoea, frequency of urination

---

MANAGEMENT OF PANIC

1 Move casualty to a quiet place.

2 Calm casualty by attentive listening, helping them relax, and encouraging them to slow breathing in unison with your own.

3 Stay with casualty until medical aid arrives.

DEPRESSION AND SUICIDAL BEHAVIOUR

Signs and symptoms

▶ sadness, dejection, self-blame, hopelessness, suicidal ideas, attempted suicide

▶ slow movements, decreased or increased appetite, weight loss or gain, insomnia, loss of interest in activities

▶ sudden dramatic change from sadness, hopelessness etc. to apparent resolution and happiness may be a sign of impending suicide

---

MANAGEMENT OF DEPRESSION AND SUICIDAL BEHAVIOUR

1 If situation is life-threatening or dangerous, have someone ☏ *call 000 for emergency services.*

2 Identify yourself as a first aider.

3 Check vital signs, if the casualty gives you permission.

4 Check level of consciousness (ask name, address, date, whereabouts).

5 Encourage the casualty to talk. Listen and remain open. Be polite and respectful.

6 Attempt to ascertain whether casualty has suicidal ideas or has taken an overdose.

7 Stay with casualty until help arrives.

THOUGHT-DISORDER

Most people with severe mental illness are not violent. They are more likely to be confused, wandering, out-of-touch, or withdrawn.

Signs and symptoms

- disorganised thinking, racing thoughts, emotions not consistent with thinking
- hearing or seeing things that aren't there
- odd or false ideas (e.g. that some group or person is following them)

MANAGEMENT OF THOUGHT-DISORDER

1 ☎ *Call 000 for emergency services.*

2 Approach casualty quietly. Identify yourself as a first aider.

3 Be polite and respectful. Stay calm, yet firm and in control. Reassure casualty that help is on the way.

4 Ask permission to monitor vital signs.

5 Check level of consciousness (ask name, address, date, whereabouts).

6 Encourage casualty to talk. Listen attentively.

7 Don't interrupt, contradict or debate casualty's ideas.

8 Stay with casualty until help arrives.

VIOLENCE

Violent behaviour can result from a number of factors, or a combination of any of these: intoxication from alcohol or drugs; a mental illness in which the casualty fears attack and acts in self-defence; domestic disputes; physical illness (e.g. low blood sugar).

Signs and symptoms

▶ defensive, excited, threatening, belligerent, argumentative
▶ may have a weapon
▶ may appear intoxicated
▶ shouting and talking to unseen images, etc.

MANAGEMENT OF VIOLENCE

1 ☎ *Call 000 for emergency services.*

2 Don't put yourself in danger. Protect others from getting hurt. Don't approach the casualty unless you judge it is safe. Don't approach a casualty who has a weapon. Never try to wrest a weapon from a casualty.

3 If you decide it is safe, approach casualty slowly from the front. Avoid staring at or towering over the casualty. Sit down if you think it is safe.

4 Speak gently. Identify yourself as a first aider. Encourage the casualty to talk. Be polite and respectful.

5 Check vital signs if casualty gives you permission.

6 Check casualty's level of consciousness (ask name, address, date, whereabouts).

7 Try to ascertain source of casualty's anger. Fear, grief, humiliation, rejection or depression may be at the root of the problem.

8 Stay with casualty until help arrives.

Drug and alcohol misuse

24

Drug and alcohol misuse or abuse are forms of poisoning. The personal and social costs are enormous: disability, loss of good health and even life, increased health care costs, and loss of working days and productivity.

Legal and illegal drugs are implicated in a significant number of hospital admissions, arrests, child abuse cases, suicides, road accident deaths, assaults, domestic violence, family disruption and crime.

Illnesses range from ruptured stomach linings and peptic ulcers to heart disease, liver cancer and brain damage.

Deaths may often be reported as suicide, a car accident or poisoning even when they are drug-related. Sometimes these deaths are intentional, but many are not.

This chapter discusses management of casualties suffering effects of drug misuse and abuse, the signs and symptoms of their use and the associated health costs.

Drug Use, Dependence and Addiction

The term 'drug' describes certain substances which, when taken into the body, cause some specific or abnormal physical or mental change. They are swallowed or injected for many reasons: for pain relief, to promote recovery from an illness, for some other medicinal purpose, for pleasure, for peer group approval, and for escape from problems. Drugs include legal substances such as alcohol, tobacco, and prescribed and over-the-counter medication, as well as those which are illegal.

Whether the drug is legal or illegal, its use can lead to dependency and addiction. The more a person takes of some substances, the less are the effects on the body, so the body builds up a **tolerance** to them.

A person is **dependent** on a drug when the drug is needed for normal functioning (e.g. insulin for a diabetic), or when the person feels it is needed.

Those with a dependence on a substance who develop an overwhelming and uncontrollable physical or psychological craving for it, have become **addicted**.

When an addict who has been using a drug stops using it, **withdrawal** can occur. This can cause severe mental and physical distress, including such symptoms as irritability, aggression, anger and restlessness. Some people may have seizures (fits), depending on the substance.

EFFECTS OF DRUG MISUSE AND ABUSE

Drug misuse may be:
- ▶ accidental (e.g. taking too much of a drug or the wrong dose)
- ▶ deliberate (e.g. for social or emotional reasons or with suicidal intent)

Accidental drug misuse

A person may accidentally misuse a drug when:
- ▶ too much is taken (overdose)
- ▶ taking of a dose is forgotten so another is taken
- ▶ two drugs are taken which interact to produce unintended harmful effects

The effects of accidental misuse range from not very serious to life-threatening. **Side effects** or unintended effects from a drug (e.g. diarrhoea, nausea) may result from a sensitivity to the drug.

People most at risk of accidental drug misuse

- ▶ those who regularly take a number of medications
- ▶ those who take other people's medication
- ▶ those who experiment with drugs
- ▶ children (due to curiosity or mistaking medication for lolly or cordial)
- ▶ the elderly

People may take multiple doses of their medication if they become confused. This is more likely to happen if:
- ▶ the person is on a number of drugs
- ▶ containers or medication are changed
- ▶ directions are not detailed or clear
- ▶ the person is not aware what condition the medication is for

Deliberate drug misuse and abuse

In Australia, the most misused and abused substances are alcohol and tobacco. Although the initial effects of these social drugs are usually pleasurable, there are dangers associated with their use. Pharmaceuticals may be misused, for example when people take a cocktail of drugs with alcohol, or overuse painkillers etc.

Deliberate drug misuse can also result from suicidal intentions. The amount taken may be just enough to gain attention—a 'cry for help'—or enough to kill the person.

Effects

The immediate effects of drug misuse can be nausea, diarrhoea, vomiting, depressed breathing, irregular heartbeat and unconsciousness. The longer-term effects can be damage to the kidneys, liver, lungs and brain.

The wider impact of drugs includes social effects such as accidents (e.g. drowning, car accidents), aggression, violence, family disruption, absenteeism, and theft to maintain a drug habit.

RISK MANAGEMENT

Casualties who are under the influence of drugs or alcohol may be at risk of harming themselves or others through dangerous or violent behaviour. In handling such a situation:

▶ **DO NOT** put yourself at risk
▶ **DO NOT** approach the casualty if you do not feel it is safe
▶ **DO NOT** be judgmental (you could provoke hostility)

MANAGEMENT OF DRUG AND ALCOHOL MISUSE

1 Follow DRABC:
> DRABC
- Danger—risk management
- Response—what is level of consciousness?
- Airway—be mindful of danger to airway from vomiting
- Breathing—consider oxygen therapy and EAR with resuscitation equipment if necessary
- Circulation—manage for shock; give CPR if necessary.

2 ☎ *Call 000 for an ambulance.*

3 Be calm, reassuring and sympathetic, and act professionally; quietly move casualty to safety if necessary.

4 Be aware of the possibility of infectious hepatitis or AIDS as a result of using contaminated needles—follow universal precautions to avoid infection (*see p. 88*).

5 Remove any weapons and potential missiles from the vicinity if possible.

6 Discreetly direct bystanders away from the scene.

7 Seek information:
- history—what, when, and how much has casualty taken or used?
- observations—monitor vital signs frequently (including conscious state).

8 Maintain an open airway—casualty may have convulsions, vomit or become unconscious.

9 Attempt to keep vomit, or at least a sample, to send with casualty to hospital.

10 Check for possible fractures or other injuries—give appropriate first aid.

11 Keep drugs or containers for identification—send with casualty to hospital.

COMMONLY MISUSED SUBSTANCES

STIMULANTS

Stimulants increase a person's feelings of excitement, energy and happiness. They affect the nervous system, speeding up mental and physical activity, making the person feel more alert and more able to perform a task.

Depending on the type of stimulant, use may be characterised by over-stimulation, exhilaration, excitability, visual disturbances, hallucinations and delusions.

Signs and symptoms

Signs of the use of stimulants may include an increase in pulse and respiration, sweating, irritability, nausea, vomiting and odd behaviour.

Stimulants may be swallowed, sniffed, injected or inhaled. They include:
- amphetamines (also called uppers, speed, ice)
- cocaine (also referred to as coke and crack)
- designer drugs such as ecstasy

Legal substances which act as stimulants, especially when overused, include:
- coffee and tea
- nicotine
- soft drinks containing caffeine

HALLUCINOGENS

Signs and symptoms

Hallucinogens cause changes in mood, emotions, sensation and self-awareness. They can alter the person's perceptions of time and space and produce delusions. During a 'bad trip', the person may feel intense fear, panic, profound depression, tension and anxiety.

The most common hallucinogens are:
- lysergic acid diethylamide (LSD or acid)
- certain types of mushrooms (e.g. gold tops)
- phencyclidine (angel dust)
- marijuana, hashish
- mescaline (peyote or buttons)

DEPRESSANTS

Depressants affect the central nervous system, slowing down mental and physical activity. They are usually swallowed as tablets, liquids or powder but may occasionally be inhaled or injected.

Signs and symptoms

The principal dangers of depressants are impairment of coordination and judgment and depression of all body functions including consciousness, heart function (or cardiac output), blood pressure and respiration. Oxygen therapy may be of particular need in first aid treatment when depressants have been misused.

Common depressants (street names—downers, reds, benzos) include:
- barbiturates, benzodiazepines
- narcotics
- alcohol
- various inhalants (e.g. petrol, thinners, glue)

PHARMACEUTICALS

Pharmaceuticals are a group of drugs with which there is an increasing problem of misuse and abuse. Casualties who have overdosed on pharmaceuticals have often taken a combination of drugs that affect their level of consciousness.

It is important to get help quickly, to try to prevent the casualty taking any more drugs, and to be ready to perform EAR or CPR if necessary, until help arrives.

PARACETAMOL

Paracetamol is currently the safest, general purpose painkiller for mild to moderate pain. Special care is needed for its use in children. There is a narrow 'window' between its effective dose and its toxic dose. Too much causes serious, potentially fatal , liver damage. DO NOT deviate from the prescribed dosage (1/2 tablet for 7-12 year old) in children. Always read the directions on the packaging before administrating this medication.

CHILDREN AND DRUG POISONING

The most common cause of poisoning in young children is swallowing medication or household products not safely stored.

MANAGEMENT OF DRUG POISONING—CHILD

1 **DO NOT** make the child vomit—this can cause further harm.

2 If the child does vomit, keep vomitus to show the doctor.

3 **DO NOT** give fluids—this will dissolve the drugs and hasten absorption.

4 ☎ *Call the Poisons Information Centre—13 11 26.*

5 Reassure the child.

6 Ask the child:
- how many pills were swallowed
- when pills were taken.

7 Seek medical aid.

If the child is unconscious:

1 ☎ *Call 000 for an ambulance.*

2 Open the child's mouth and hook out with a finger any tablets you can see.

3 Place child on side in recovery position and check ABC.

ALCOHOL POISONING IN CHILDREN

Signs and symptoms Even a small amount of alcohol can be harmful to a young child. Signs and symptoms that a child has drunk alcohol are a strong smell of alcohol; a flushed, moist face; slurred speech; staggering; deep, noisy breathing; nausea; a pounding pulse.

MANAGEMENT OF ALCOHOL POISONING—CHILD

1 Seek medical aid.

2 Allow child to rest; help lie in recovery position.

3 Examine bottle or ask child how much was drunk.

4 Place a bowl near child in case of vomiting.

5 If child goes to sleep, check they can be roused easily.

6 If child unconscious, place on side in recovery position and check ABC.

Sports injuries

Millions of Australians play some form of
sport. Most are injured at least once during
their sporting lives. A high proportion of
these injuries could have been prevented.

Injuries occur more often in some sports,
for example football, the martial arts and
netball, than in others.

This chapter covers in detail the management of injuries that are specifically caused
through participation in a sport and are
unlikely to have been caused by some
other means. The management of injuries
covered in other chapters, such as spinal
injuries in chapter eight, will not be
covered.

SPORTS INJURIES

There are approximately one million sports injuries in Australia annually. Football, netball, basketball, hockey and cricket account for 75% of injuries from organised sports and 50% of all sport and recreation injuries. Those who compete on a recreational basis at weekends are more likely to be injured than those who compete professionally or semi-professionally.

Bruising, as a result of a direct blow, is the most common form of minor sports injury, followed by strains, sprains and tearing. Knee and ankle injuries are the two most commonly treated sports injuries with 20% of knee injuries requiring surgery. Twenty per cent of ankle injuries are serious. An increasing number of injuries are a result of over-using particular parts of the body (e.g. joint or tendon pain following excessive participation in aerobic exercise).

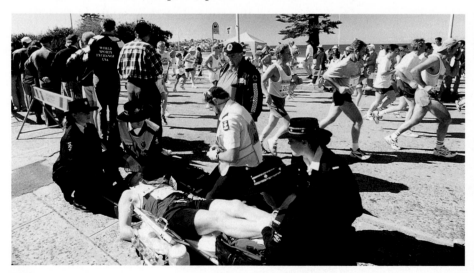

COMMON SPORTS INJURIES

Football	• corked thigh (a painful bruise to the large muscles on front of thigh as a result of a heavy blow) • head injuries (e.g. concussion) resulting from collisions • spinal cord injury (particularly in Rugby League and Rugby Union) • knee and ankle injuries (particularly in Australian Rules, soccer and touch football) • shoulder injuries
Netball and basketball	• knee, ankle and leg injuries • concussion and other head injuries resulting from collisions
Hockey	• injuries to lower limbs • injuries from being hit by stick or ball
Cricket	• injuries from being hit by bat or ball • knee and ankle injuries
Skateboards/ in-line skates/ skates	• knee, elbow and hand injuries • broken legs, ankles, sprains
Bicycles	• hand, knee injuries • head injuries
Athletics/ 'power' sports, (e.g. jumping, sprinting)	• dehydration • painful, stiff muscles
Jogging	• injuries to lower limbs • heat stress
Squash/tennis	• eye injuries

Note: Incorrect and inappropriate training as well as over-training are believed to account for 40% of all acute sports injuries.

MANAGEMENT OF SPORTS INJURIES

From the first aider's point of view, management of sports injuries is no different from that of the same injury from any other cause.

Having managed the injury, one needs to also consider whether the casualty:

▶ can continue playing
▶ should be withdrawn from play

A casualty should be advised to seek medical advice before returning to play after an injury (unless injury is minor).

When an injury has occurred and the player has received first aid, it will often be up to the casualty to ensure that ongoing management is appropriate. **It is best to avoid:**

H   Heat increases bleeding and swelling.
A   Alcohol increases bleeding and swelling.
R   Running (or exercise) too soon causes further injury.
M   Massage in the first 24–48 hours causes bleeding and swelling.

When you have to give first aid to someone with a sports injury:

▶ remember DRABC
▶ assess injuries as they occur, not at the end of the event
▶ assess the injury carefully before moving a casualty

> never move a casualty with a suspected spinal injury—wait for medical aid
> remember RICE (Rest, Ice, Compression, Elevation, *see p.122*)

The sports injuries described in this chapter are listed in alphabetical order for easy reference.

ABDOMINAL INJURIES

Abdominal injuries are rare in sports but can be caused by a blow to the abdomen or by impact from an object at high speed (e.g. in surfing).

There is the possibility of internal bleeding as the vital organs (spleen, kidneys and liver) can be injured.

MANAGEMENT OF ABDOMINAL INJURIES

1 Follow DRABC.

2 Check for signs of internal bleeding (*see p. 117*).

3 If abdominal pain continues, seek medical aid immediately.

AIR PRESSURE INJURIES

Air pressure changes that occur during scuba diving can result in life-threatening injury. Such injuries can be prevented by adequate preparation and training, and adherence to safety procedures.

Common injuries are:
> ruptured eardrum
> acute facial pain
> decompression sickness or 'the bends' (due to

    nitrogen bubbles forming in the blood)—can
    be life-threatening

▶   rupture of air sacs of the lungs

▶   arterial gas embolism (air bubbles forming in
    the blood as a result of a ruptured lung)—this
    can be life-threatening

MANAGEMENT OF INJURIES CAUSED BY AIR PRESSURE CHANGES

1   Follow DRABC.

2   ☎ *Call 000 for an ambulance.*

3   Give 100% oxygen if available.

4   Casualty must remain lying down (to prevent cerebral gas embolism).

5   ☎ *Call 1800 088 200 for Diving Emergency Services.*

ANKLE SPRAINS

Ankle sprains result in rupture of ligaments on either side of the joint. First aiders must be aware of the possibility that the bones of the ankle may have been fractured, although this is difficult to identify.

The injured ankle will be tender, bruised and will become swollen. Pain can be quite intense and will restrict movement and cause loss of function.

MANAGEMENT OF ANKLE SPRAINS

1   Follow RICE.

2   Manage as for a fractured ankle *(see p. 133).*

3   Seek medical aid.

CHEST INJURIES

Injuries to the rib cage commonly occur in football and surfing or by direct blows in any sport. The casualty may experience pain over the injured area, difficulty breathing and may be gasping for breath. The casualty may also cough up blood. For the management of suspected fractured ribs (see p. 146).

Over-exertion can result in a cramp (a 'stitch').

MANAGEMENT OF A 'STITCH'

1 Ask casualty to breathe slowly and deeply and to rest.

CORKED THIGH

A corked thigh is caused by a blow to the front or outer thigh muscles. It results in bleeding into the muscles, the injured area becoming tight and painful as the muscles contract. Any stretching will cause further bleeding.

MANAGEMENT OF A CORKED THIGH

1 Follow RICE.

2 Do not stretch the muscle.

3 Seek medical aid.

EYE INJURIES

Eye injuries occur most commonly when playing squash or tennis. Wearing some form of eye protection is important. All eye injuries are potentially serious and casualties should be referred immediately to medical aid. For management of eye injuries (see p. 172–3).

FINGER INJURIES

Finger injuries may occur as a result of a blow or the finger being stretched out of normal position. They often occur in hard ball or body contact sports (e.g. cricket, football, judo, boxing).

Fractured finger

For management of a fractured finger *(see p. 134)*.

Dislocated finger or thumb

A dislocated finger or thumb may be caused by over-extension, over-flexing or twisting. The joint may be partially or completely dislocated. If the finger or thumb is completely dislocated, inability to move the joint, intense pain and deformity will be obvious. If partially dislocated, deformity may not be obvious and some degree of movement may be possible.

MANAGEMENT OF DISLOCATED FINGER OR THUMB

1 Elevate the hand.

2 **DO NOT** attempt to put finger or thumb back in place.

3 Strap to adjoining finger as a splint.

4 Seek medical aid.

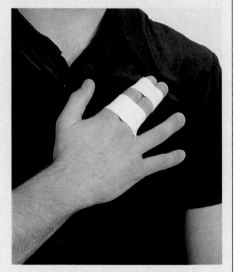

Mallet finger

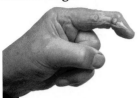

This is a deformity of the finger due to a rupture of the tendon or a chip fracture of the base of the end bone near the joint. The finger will be painful, swollen and tender and the casualty will not be able to extend the finger from a flexed position.

MANAGEMENT OF A MALLET FINGER

1 **DO NOT** straighten finger.

2 Immobilise and place splint on finger.

3 Seek medical aid.

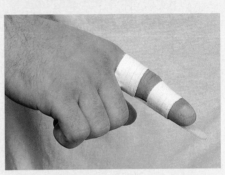

Contusions of the fingernail or toenail

Contusions may occur under a fingernail or toenail when blood collects beneath it following a blow or crush injury. The end of the finger will be painful and throbbing, blood will collect beneath the nail and the fingertip will be tender.

MANAGEMENT OF FINGERNAIL OR TOENAIL CONTUSIONS

1 Apply icepacks.

2 Seek medical aid.

FRACTURED NOSE

A fractured nose commonly occurs in contact sports such as football, boxing and martial arts and is usually accompanied by bleeding.

MANAGEMENT OF A FRACTURED NOSE

1 Manage bleeding—sit casualty forward; apply icepacks to neck and forehead.

2 Seek medical aid.

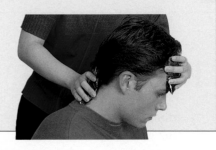

GROIN AND TESTICLE INJURIES

Injuries to the groin and testicles can occur as a result of a direct blow or in the case of groin injuries, by overstretching muscles of the groin or upper thigh. The injury will be associated with severe pain. The testicles should be protected if playing sports which use a hard ball (e.g. cricket).

MANAGEMENT OF GROIN AND TESTICLE INJURIES

1 Follow DRABC.

2 Lie casualty on back with knees slightly bent and supported by a folded blanket or in a position of comfort.

3 Apply icepacks for groin injury.

4 Rest and reassure casualty.

5 Seek medical aid.

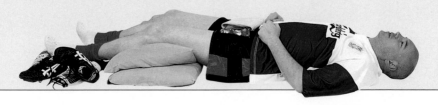

HEAD AND FACIAL INJURIES

Head and facial injuries commonly occur in vehicular sports and those where there is body contact (e.g. football), especially if a faceguard or mouthguard is not worn. Facial injuries may involve the eyes, nose and teeth, and may include facial lacerations and fractures. For management of head injuries *(see p. 159)*. For management of other facial injuries *(see p. 106–10)*.

KNEE INJURIES

Knee injuries are common in sport. Immediate first aid limits swelling and shortens recovery time.

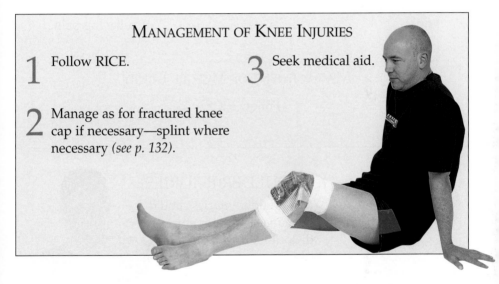

MANAGEMENT OF KNEE INJURIES

1 Follow RICE.

2 Manage as for fractured knee cap if necessary—splint where necessary *(see p. 132)*.

3 Seek medical aid.

MUSCLE CRAMP AND INJURIES

Cramps are spasms or abnormal contractions of muscles. The causes are varied, including overuse, excessive jarring, a small tear, loss of body salts and fluids as a result of excessive sweating, or poor blood supply to the area (e.g. because clothing is too tight).

The casualty may feel pain, be unable to use the cramped muscle and the muscle may stiffen as it shortens and contracts.

A muscle injury will occur when a muscle is stretched beyond its normal limit. This can result in a stretched or torn muscle. When a muscle is injured in this way, it is important to prevent swelling in order to promote recovery.

MANAGEMENT OF MUSCLE CRAMP

1 Gently stretch the affected muscle fully.

2 Apply icepacks.

3 Massage gently, if this assists in relieving pain.

MANAGEMENT OF MUSCLE INJURY

1 Follow RICE.

SHOULDER INJURIES

All shoulder injuries should be managed as a fracture or dislocation *(see p. 133–6).*

SOFT TISSUE INJURIES OF THE NECK

These injuries are often associated with bruising. Swelling can result in airway obstruction, leading to a lack of oxygen, unconsciousness and death.

MANAGEMENT OF SOFT TISSUE INJURIES TO THE NECK

1 Follow DRABC.

2 If casualty conscious:
   • loosen clothing around neck
   • apply icepacks to neck.

3 Support neck using a cervical collar, firmly rolled towel or a padded roll of newspaper.

4 Observe casualty carefully for airway problems or signs of internal bleeding.

5 ☎ *Call 000 for an ambulance.*

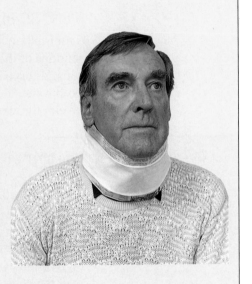

SPINAL INJURIES

These occur, fortunately rarely, in body contact sports such as football, and in diving or surfing. A casualty with a spinal injury should only be moved in exceptional circumstances such as when there is serious danger or possible further injury may occur. In such circumstances, great care should be taken and the proper equipment used if available. A scoop stretcher, Jordon frame or similar are appropriate. For management of spinal injuries *(see p. 162)*.

STRESS FRACTURES

Repetitive overuse can cause a stress fracture, which is a breakdown within the interior of the bone. This sort of injury most commonly occurs in the long bones of the foot and in the kneecap. Signs and symptoms are pain and tenderness at the site. Management of a stress fracture is the same as for other fractures *(see p. 133)*.

TENNIS ELBOW

Tennis elbow is a strain of the muscles and tendons of the elbow as a result of overuse. The muscles become overstressed and the injury may be chronic. It occurs in many sports (e.g. tennis, javelin throwing and baseball).

MANAGEMENT OF TENNIS ELBOW

1 Apply icepacks to the elbow.

2 Rest the arm in a sling.

3 Seek medical aid.

Signs and symptoms include pain and tenderness over the bone at the side of the elbow joint (usually on the outer side) which is made worse by contracting or stretching the muscles attached to that joint.

'WINDING'

'Winding' or 'being winded' usually results from a blow to the abdomen, or from a fall. The casualty usually gasps and tries to breathe. The mouth is wide open but the chest does not move air in or out.

MANAGEMENT OF 'WINDING'

1 Rest and reassure casualty.

2 Place casualty in a comfortable position that assists breathing.

3 Do not pump legs or massage abdominal wall (this may cause further damage if seriously injured).

4 Seek medical aid if the casualty does not improve within a few minutes.

BLISTERS

Blisters are caused by excessive friction to the skin, and usually occur during sporting/recreational activities such as hiking, running, jogging, and fun runs. If friction is felt, stop activity and tape the exposed area to avoid blisters forming.

MANAGEMENT OF BLISTERS

1 Put on protective gloves—to minimize infection.

2 Puncture edge of blister at 3 or 4 points with a cleaned needle.

3 Gently express fluid—do not remove skin covering blister.

4 Cover with a sterile transparent or non-adhesive dressing.

5 Apply padding and tape.

6 If the area becomes reddened, feels warm or painful—seek medical aid.

Focus on Safety

It has been estimated that 30% of all sports injuries can be prevented. This includes 90% of chronic injuries and 25% of acute injuries. Experts say the greatest potential for injury prevention is in:

- education of coaches and trainers
- more adequate preparation and training by players and participants
- warm-ups before sports activities
- greater use of protective gear (e.g. helmets, shin pads, eye protection)
- wearing appropriate footwear (particularly in such sports as netball and basketball)

- ensuring sporting facilities, particularly ground surfaces, are of a good standard, with padding of goal posts and other hard objects or surfaces
- modifying and changing rules which contribute to injuries
- recognising concussion and not permitting players to resume competition until it is safe to do so

Other preventive measures include ensuring that all sportspeople:

- are playing at the appropriate standard
- do not resume sport until fully recovered from an injury

Remote area first aid

CONTENTS

Much of Australia is made up of remote and wilderness areas. The Australian outback, alpine wilderness and the many national parks all pose particular challenges to those dealing with an injured person. A knowledge of first aid and a readiness to be self-reliant will give confidence to all who live, work or travel in these areas.

Being able to manage injuries in a remote area in a skilled and confident manner may save a life. Help may be delayed— for a day or more—and transporting the injured to medical assistance can be a prolonged process. In such circumstances, skilled first aid can prevent complications and help with a speedy recovery.

This chapter briefly outlines what has to be considered in managing a sick or injured person in a remote area: how to monitor vital signs; fluid intake and output; bandages, dressings and splints; hygiene, toileting and protection from the elements.

REMOTE AREA FIRST AID

A remote area is defined as one where access to medical assistance is hampered by time and distance. This includes not only outback areas but also national parks, bushland, wilderness or mountain areas, and the sea. In any of these areas it may take some hours or even days to reach, or be reached by, emergency services.

Weather conditions, fires and floods can delay access to medical assistance. In remote areas, medical, nursing and ambulance personnel are few in number and may be committed in other areas at the time of need. However, every effort should be made through the use of cellular or satellite telephones, or portable two-way radios, to establish a communication link to a medical facility. If you are able to establish a link, expert advice will be available, even in the most remote areas, to help you manage the casualty. This contact will also facilitate the pick up and transport of the casualty.

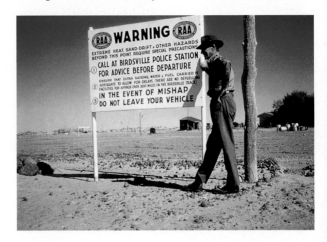

MANAGEMENT CONSIDERATIONS

The principles of first aid are always the same, in remote areas or anywhere else. However a knowledge of survival techniques and procedures for contacting medical assistance become especially important in remote areas. Consideration will also have to be given to the following points.

Whether to continue an activity
The first aider will have to decide whether a casualty can continue with work or recreational activity or whether the activity should be abandoned to take the casualty to medical aid.

Whether to travel to medical assistance or to wait for it to come
This will be influenced by such factors as the severity of the injury, the time required for medical aid to arrive, the risk that moving might hinder rescue efforts, whether the casualty can be moved safely, the safety of the location and the adequacy or otherwise of food and water supplies.

Reassurance
The casualty can become more stressed because of the longer wait for medical assistance and may need greater emotional support and reassurance. Remaining calm and regularly monitoring the casualty's condition will help reduce both the casualty's and the first aider's anxieties.

The casualty's comfort
Because of time delays, it is important to ensure the casualty is comfortable. The casualty's

conscious state and nature of injuries will determine the most comfortable position.

Documentation
A casualty's condition often changes; observing and recording changes are particularly significant—documenting everything (changes in symptoms, vital signs and first aid management) is important and can be very helpful in later treatment.

The need to monitor fluid intake and output
Dehydration can be of particular concern in a hot environment.

Shelter and survival
There is a great need to ensure the casualty is sheltered from the elements. If in a cold climate, keep the casualty warm and dry with added clothing, blankets, papers or any other materials that will help insulate the body. If in a hot climate, keep the casualty in the shade and out of direct sun, loosen clothing and wipe casualty with a wet cloth if possible. Do not forget to provide for your own shelter.

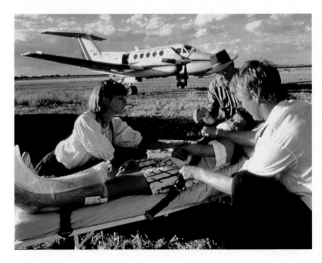

Shock
The longer a sick or injured casualty remains without medical treatment, the greater the potential for shock. Prevention and management of shock are crucial.

The need to perform a procedure for which you are not trained

You may have to perform a procedure which is beyond your training (e.g. an injection), with telephone or radio instructions from emergency services, the Royal Flying Doctor Service or a medical practitioner.

CASUALTY CARE

Observing and recording the casualty's condition

In a remote area it may be necessary to observe a casualty for a prolonged time. The type of observations will be determined by the casualty's condition and injuries. For example, a simple lower limb fracture does not usually require you to note the conscious state, pulse, breathing and pupil changes. However, it could be vital to observe and record colour and condition of the toes on the injured limb.

Remember that a casualty's condition can deteriorate. Close observation of the casualty will help early recognition of any changes and assist in further management. The recording and transmitting of such changes are of great help to rescue services.

It is particularly important to record initial observations. For a severely injured casualty, observations should be made every 30 minutes; for a less seriously injured casualty, observations may be made at hourly intervals.

Observe and regularly record the casualty's:
- ▶ **conscious state** (especially time of any changes)
  - • has it improved or deteriorated?
- ▶ **pulse** (count rate over 1 minute and record)
  - • is rate fast or slow?
  - • is rhythm regular or irregular?
  - • is it weak or strong?
- ▶ **breathing** (count rate over 1 minute and record)
  - • is rate fast or slow?

OBSERVATION CHART

Day/Date	Time	Conscious state	Pulse	Breathing	Temperature	Pupils	Skin colour	Skin conditions	Speech	Fluid intake	Fluid output	Comments

- is it deep, shallow or sighing?
- is it noisy, quiet or gurgling?
▶ **temperature** (especially any changes)
  - is it normal?
  - is it above/below 37°C?
▶ **pupils** (especially time of any changes)
  - are they dilated or contracted?
  - are they equal or unequal?
  - do they react to light?
▶ **skin colour**
  - is it normal or pale?
  - is it bluish or purplish?
▶ **skin condition**
  - is it wet or dry?
  - is it warm or cold?
▶ **speech**
  - is it slurred?
▶ **fluid intake andoutput** *(see p. 431)*

Take care if discussing casualty—don't assume casualty cannot hear or understand you even if apparently unconscious.

Managing illnesses and injuries

In a remote area, control of blood loss and infection can be more demanding, for example because blood loss may continue over a long time. Management may need to be modified depending on supplies on hand. For example the number of dressings available will dictate the number of dressing changes.

A first aider will also have to decide the seriousness of an injury to determine how urgently medical assistance is required. Is there damage to underlying body structures? How much damage is there? Is shock likely?

All wounds can become infected. When dirt and debris enter and remain in penetrating or deep wounds, infection always occurs. Such wounds need to be attended to urgently. Superficial wounds can also become infected. Abrasions can be dangerous when they involve large areas of the body, because of the risk of infection and shock. Ensure any wound is kept clean and, if wound is open, cover with a dressing. An infected wound is painful and debilitating and prolongs recovery.

CHECKING ADEQUACY OF DRESSINGS, BANDAGES AND SPLINTS

1 Inspect dressings to see whether blood has soaked through:
- add further dressings if necessary
- make sure dressings are sufficiently tight.

2 Check any fracture immobilisation for firmness of bandages:

- if loosened, apply a firm bandage over initial bandage.

3 Check circulation of limb:
- impaired if fingers or toes are pale, painful, or cold and numb; remove bandage and reapply.

Moving a casualty

In remote areas a seriously injured casualty should not be moved unless necessary. The casualty must be moved if:

▶ in danger from storms, lightning, flood or fire
▶ you decide the benefits outweigh the destabilisation movement might produce

Local movement can be needed for comfort: there may be snakes, ants or other creatures that could cause further problems, discomfort or fear; the ground may be cold; or the place where the accident occurred could be dangerous (e.g. on a narrow ledge), uncomfortable, exposed or inaccessible.

If you have to transport the casualty in a private vehicle, it is important to remain calm, and to drive at a safe speed. No matter how serious the injury or the circumstances, excessive speed will only endanger yourself and the casualty, and aggravate injuries.

Improvisation

The ability to improvise and to use whatever resources are available is a valuable skill for the first aider.

Clothing and other items may be used to control bleeding, to tie and support fractures and to pad injured parts of the body. For example:

- tea towels, socks, pillowcases, a sheet or torn piece of clothing can control bleeding or be used as dressings
- singlets, folded shirts, blouses and trousers can make padding or, if twisted tightly round and round, a ring pad around a foreign object
- shoelaces can tie padding to a splint
- shirts, singlets and blouses can be cut into strips for roller bandages
- long socks, long sleeves or clothing cut into 10 cm strips can make collar and cuff slings
- coats and jackets with poles passed through sleeves can make stretchers

Other items can also be used: sacks and sleeping bags with poles passed through them can be used as stretchers, as can flat pieces of strong material (e.g. lengths of timber, door, side panel of a vehicle); tree branches can be used as splints or poles; folded newspaper can be used as a splint or neck collar.

Toiletting hygiene and comfort

The mobile casualty can use a latrine dug in the ground. However, if the casualty is not mobile, a billy can, water bottle, plastic bag or other container can be used as an improvised urinal. For

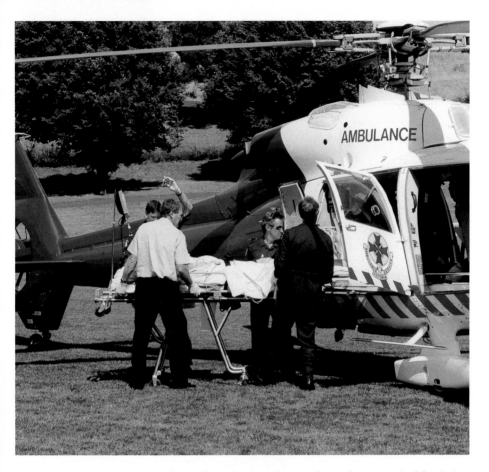

bowel motions, a large plastic bag is suitable. It is essential the casualty's hands are washed after toileting and that waste is buried in a deep pit. Handwashing and infection control procedures should be followed whenever possible.

Fluid intake and output

When evacuation may be delayed for some time, it is necessary to ensure the casualty maintains an adequate fluid intake to prevent dehydration. However, the amount of fluid given will be determined by the type and extent of the casualty's injuries and level of consciousness.

431

Casualties not severely injured may eat and drink as usual. But if a casualty shows signs and symptoms of shock, and if you are more than three hours from help, you should give clear fluids or ice cubes to suck if the casualty can take them. If the casualty, especially a child, has diarrhoea, give as much fluid as the casualty wants. Frequent small amounts are best.
Oral rehydration salts, made up with water, are ideal and should be carried by all who venture into the outback and other remote areas.

Casualties who have abdominal pain, a reduced level of consciousness or who cannot pass urine should not usually be given any fluids, or only sips at the most. However, mouth and lip care are important—wipe face and lips and apply lanolin cream as lip balm if available.

For other casualties:
- moisten casualty's lips with water for the first 4–8 hours after injury
- give small amounts of water e.g. 100 mls/half a cup every half hour if medical aid has not arrived after 4–8 hours
- stop giving water if the casualty vomits or shows other signs of discomfort
- if surgical care is likely within 4–6 hours, do not give food or drink to a casualty whose condition is serious, for example severe open fractures, internal injuries, and fractures that involve other organs (e.g. skull and pelvic fractures)

It is necessary to monitor fluid intake and output when the casualty:
- drinks water
- vomits

▶ passes urine
▶ loses blood
▶ develops diarrhoea

Where possible, the volume should be recorded using a convenient measure such as a cup or soup tin. The measuring device should be kept with the casualty and shown to medical personnel.
Blood, vomit, faeces and excessive sweating can be difficult to measure and may simply be recorded as being 'small', 'moderate' or 'large'. The time should also be recorded. Note whether urine is concentrated or odourless and whether blood (smokiness) is present.

General nursing care

A casualty who lies immobile for long periods of time may develop reddened pressure areas over bony prominences such as heels, buttocks, and shoulderblades. Facial areas such as ears are of particular concern. Circulation becomes impaired to skin areas that remain in contact with hard surfaces (such as the ground). These areas need to be relieved of pressure using padding.

Turn the casualty every 3–4 hours. Turn more frequently if skin becomes damaged and a sore develops. Care for all unconscious casualties in the recovery position.

If two or more persons are present with a casualty in a remote area, and one has to leave to summon help, the general rule is that the most experienced first aider remains with the casualty.

Chapter

27

How the body functions

The body is made up of a number of systems, organs and other structures. Each has a function to perform, but none works independently.

This chapter outlines the functions of each system and the role of the major associated organs.

The skeleton, which is the body's supporting structure, is also described.

THE BODY'S SYSTEMS

The body is made up of systems which have different functions to perform in keeping the body alive and well. These systems are described below.

Circulatory system

The circulatory system comprises the heart, blood and blood vessels (veins, arteries and capillaries). It keeps all parts of the body supplied with oxygen-rich blood and the various sugars, proteins, vitamins, minerals and hormones needed for growth and health. This system also transports carbon dioxide, urea and other waste products to be eliminated.

Respiratory system

The respiratory system includes the lungs, wind-pipe or trachea (airway from larynx to lungs), bronchi (two tubes branching off trachea), bronchioles (smaller tubes branching off bronchi), millions of alveoli (air sacs), and diaphragm (a smooth flat muscle under the lungs). This system keeps the body supplied with oxygen and removes carbon dioxide.

Digestive and urinary systems

The digestive and urinary systems are made up of the oesophagus (gullet), stomach, liver, kidneys, gall bladder, pancreas, small and large intestines, rectum, bladder and urethra. These systems have two main functions—to convert food to simpler substances and a finer consistency so it can be absorbed into the blood and taken to all parts of the body; and to eliminate waste products.

Nervous system

The nervous system includes the brain, the spinal cord and the network of nerves which go to every part of the body. This system transports information, using electrical impulses and chemicals, from one part of the body to another.

Lymphatic system

The lymphatic system includes lymph, lymph vessels, lymph nodes and the spleen. It is responsible for transporting lymph, a fluid containing white cells used in the fight against infection.

Musculoskeletal system

The musculoskeletal system consists of the bones, muscles, ligaments and tendons which support the body, protect the internal organs and allow the various parts of the body to move *(see p. 124 for detail)*.

BODY SYSTEMS

SYSTEM	MAJOR ORGANS	MAJOR FUNCTIONS
Circulatory	heart, blood, blood vessels	• transports nutrients and oxygen • removes waste products
Respiratory	airway, lungs	• supplies oxygen • removes waste gases
Digestive and urinary	stomach, intestines, pancreas, rectum, kidneys, bladder, urethra	• converts food and liquids into proteins, sugars and other substances • collects and eliminates waste products
Nervous	brain, spinal cord, nerves	• transmits messages to and from brain
Lymphatic	lymph, lymph nodes, spleen	• fights infection
Musculo-skeletal	bones, ligaments, muscles, tendons	• provides body's framework • protects internal organs • provides the mechanical basis for movement

CIRCULATORY SYSTEM

The circulatory system is a complex circuit which enables blood to circulate throughout the entire body, transporting oxygen and nutrients to every cell and collecting waste products for elimination from the body.

The heart provides the pumping action needed to keep blood flowing throughout the body. The heart is a muscular organ the size of a clenched fist which acts as a two-sided pump, first relaxing and filling up with blood and then contracting to squeeze (or pump) the blood out into the blood vessels. This pumping action is automatic and is controlled by a complex system of nerves.

Blood

Blood is made up of:
- ▶ **plasma**—pale yellow liquid in which blood cells are suspended; contains proteins, electrolytes and various nutrients; is capable of clotting
- ▶ **red blood cells**—carry oxygen
- ▶ **white blood cells**—protect body from germs
- ▶ **platelets**—form clots to stop bleeding

Pulse

The heart's contractions can be felt in the arteries close to the skin, primarily at the neck (carotid artery), wrist (radial artery) and groin (femoral artery). The beat felt with each contraction is called a pulse.

Blood vessels

Arteries are large, strong blood vessels which carry oxygen-rich blood to all parts of the body. They subdivide into smaller blood vessels then capillaries—tiny, thin-walled blood vessels which

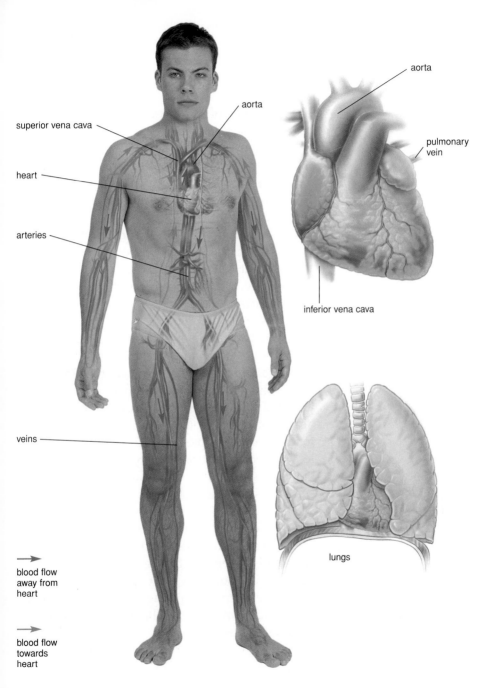

aorta

superior vena cava

aorta

heart

pulmonary vein

arteries

inferior vena cava

veins

→ blood flow away from heart

→ blood flow towards heart

lungs

439

transport blood to all cells of the body. After the cells receive oxygen from the blood, veins carry the blood, now low in oxygen, to the heart and then to the lungs.

Circulation

The circulation of blood begins and ends at the heart and consists of:

▶   **pulmonary circulation**—starting on the right side of the heart, blood is pumped to the lungs where it loses carbon dioxide and absorbs oxygen, and then goes back to the left side of the heart

▶   **systemic circulation**—starting on the left side of the heart, blood is pumped to the body, where it delivers oxygen and removes carbon dioxide, and then returns to the right side of the heart

Effects of bleeding

If an injury results in external or internal bleeding, the body tries to minimise blood loss. When a blood vessel is damaged, it will contract to slow or stop blood loss through the wound, and clots form to further restrict the bleeding. If bleeding is heavy, the contraction of blood vessels also helps to maintain blood pressure. With continued blood loss, the body has trouble compensating and blood pressure drops. The casualty then starts showing signs of shock.

Body tissues that do not receive enough oxygen can be permanently damaged or die. If an artery supplying the brain is blocked, brain cells die, resulting in a stroke. A heart attack occurs when one of the arteries supplying the heart with blood is blocked. Some muscle cells die, leading to damaged heart muscle.

RESPIRATORY SYSTEM

The body needs a constant supply of oxygen to function and survive. When a person breathes in (inhales), air is taken into the air sacs of the lungs where oxygen crosses to the blood to be transported to all parts of the body. The blood also brings carbon dioxide and other waste gases from around the body to the lungs where it crosses to the air sacs. This waste is then forced from the body when a person breathes out (exhales).

Inhaled air contains 21% oxygen while exhaled air contains about 16% oxygen and more carbon dioxide than inhaled air. (The 16% oxygen in exhaled breath is more than enough to give to a non-breathing casualty during CPR.)

Mechanics of breathing

The diaphragm and the muscles between the ribs (intercostals) work together to expand the chest. When the chest expands, air is pulled into the lungs. As these muscles relax, the chest returns to its usual size and the air is forced out. It is possible to use extra muscles in the neck and shoulders to increase force and rate of breathing. These are used as a result of heavy exercise or when a person is suffering from chest disease.

Inhalation

Air is breathed in through the mouth or nose and passes down the trachea to the two bronchi which take the air into the lungs. The bronchi then branch further into a number of smaller tubes called bronchioles which end in millions of tiny air sacs called alveoli. The walls of the alveoli and capillaries are thin so that oxygen and carbon dioxide cross through them. Thus oxygen enters the blood and carbon dioxide enters the alveoli.

Oxygen/carbon dioxide balance

The part of the brain which controls respiration monitors the amount of oxygen and carbon dioxide in the blood and responds to changes in these levels by changing the rate and depth of breathing. The amount of oxygen being used by the body is related to the amount of physical activity. The more energetic the activity, the greater the amount of oxygen required and the more carbon dioxide produced. Fever and illness may also increase demands for oxygen.

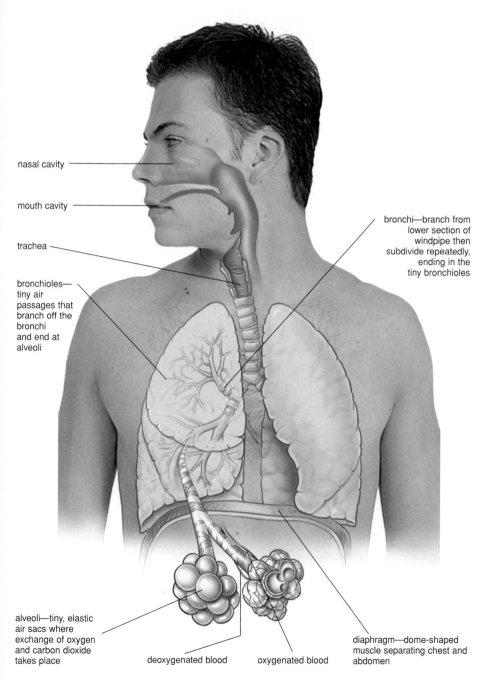

nasal cavity

mouth cavity

trachea

bronchioles—tiny air passages that branch off the bronchi and end at alveoli

bronchi—branch from lower section of windpipe then subdivide repeatedly, ending in the tiny bronchioles

alveoli—tiny, elastic air sacs where exchange of oxygen and carbon dioxide takes place

deoxygenated blood

oxygenated blood

diaphragm—dome-shaped muscle separating chest and abdomen

Digestive and Urinary Systems

The digestive system converts food and liquid into nutrients to keep the cells functioning. It also removes waste products.

Food moves from the mouth, where saliva has begun the process of breaking the food down, through the oesophagus to the stomach where it is partly digested by gastric juices. As the food is expelled from the stomach it is mixed with other digestive juices from the pancreas (insulin), liver and gall bladder. These juices help to break down the complex structure of the food into simpler forms. Insulin helps control blood sugar levels.

The food then moves on to the small intestine where the digestive process is completed and the nutrients are absorbed into the blood. The material left after this process moves to the large intestine and is eliminated from the rectum as faeces.

Urinary system

Other waste products are extracted from the blood by the kidneys which produce between one and two litres of urine daily. This moves down the ureter to the bladder, where it is held until it is voided through the urethra.

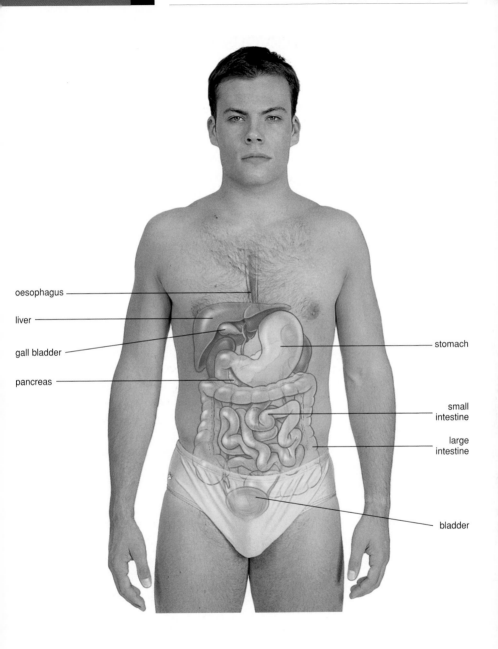

oesophagus

liver

gall bladder

pancreas

stomach

small
intestine

large
intestine

bladder

Nervous System

The nervous system is made up of the brain, spinal cord and nerves.

Brain

The brain is the controlling organ of the body and regulates all body functions. Through the body's network of nerves, the brain receives and transmits information as electrical impulses and chemicals.

Sensory and motor nerves

Sensory nerves, which transmit impulses from the body to the brain, relay information about touch, sight, sound, smell, taste, spatial awareness and pain. Motor nerves control movement by initiating muscle contraction.

Spinal cord

The spinal cord is a large group of nerves which extends from the brain down the backbone through a canal in the spine. Nerves extend from the brain and the spinal cord to every part of the body. At each vertebra of the spinal cord, two nerves branch out, one to each side of the body. In the upper part of the spinal cord, just below the brain, are the automatic centres for breathing and heart control.

Voluntary and autonomic systems

The voluntary nervous system controls the functions directed by the conscious mind, for example walking, running, eating. The autonomic nervous system controls involuntary functions such as heartbeat, breathing, digestion and blood pressure.

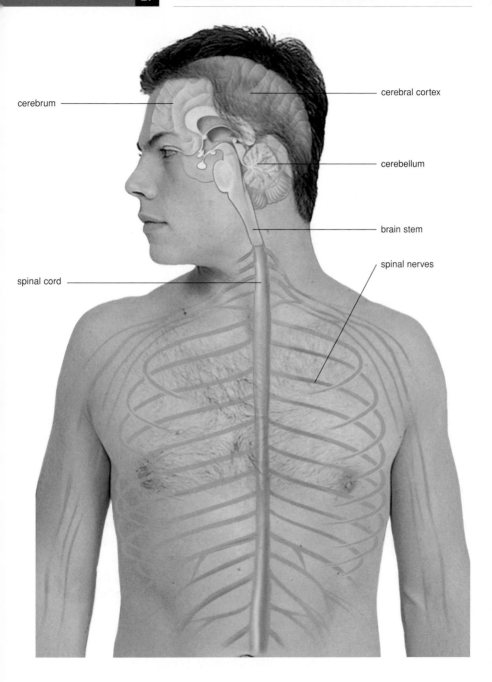

cerebrum

cerebral cortex

cerebellum

brain stem

spinal nerves

spinal cord

Lymphatic System

The lymphatic vessels pick up fluid that has been left behind in the tissues by the circulatory system and transports it back to the main veins just before they reach the heart. The lymphatic vessels come from all over the body, and contain one-way valves, so that the fluid they carry flows only towards the heart. This fluid (lymph) contains white blood cells, giving the lymphatic system a role in fighting infection.

Lymph nodes

As lymph fluid is transported towards the heart, it passes through lymph nodes (sometimes referred to as 'glands'), which contain many white cells and serve as filters. The white cells form antibodies and remove bacteria, viruses and other foreign substances. When they become activated, lymph nodes will sometimes become enlarged. This can occur before and during many common infections (e.g. influenza, glandular fever, septicaemia and skin infections). Lymph nodes may be felt in the neck, under the arm and in the groin.

White cells and spleen

White cells are found throughout the body. As well as producing antibodies and fighting infection, they have a role to play in removing and repairing old tissue, in causing fever, and in inflammation and repair of wounds. The spleen carries out these functions, as well as being a filter for the blood, and has the body's biggest concentration of white cells.

The importance of the immunity given by white blood cells is seen in conditions like AIDS,

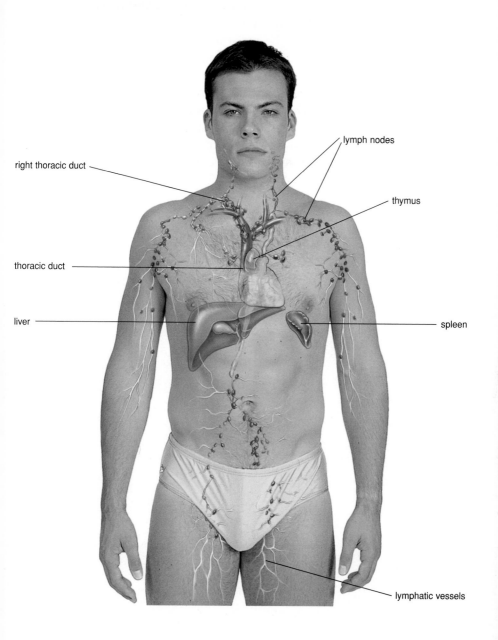

right thoracic duct

lymph nodes

thymus

thoracic duct

liver

spleen

lymphatic vessels

in which the white cells are destroyed slowly by the human immunodeficiency virus (HIV) and the body becomes susceptible to many infections that would not normally cause illness.

Lymph vessels and toxins

The lymphatic vessels provide the major route by which many venomous toxins enter the circulatory system. By using the pressure immobilisation bandage and keeping a limb still by splinting, it is possible to slow or even stop lymph fluid entering the circulation.

Musculoskeletal System

The musculoskeletal system is made up of various bones, muscles, tendons, ligaments and joints. It provides support for the body, gives protection to internal organs, stores minerals, produces blood cells in the marrow and makes movement possible.

The skeleton is the supporting structure that gives the body its general shape and provides a strong framework to which muscles are attached *(see p. 125)*. It also protects many of the organs—for example, the brain is protected by the skull, the heart and lungs by the rib cage, and the spinal cord by the vertebrae of the spine.

MAIN BONES OF THE SKELETON

Bones

Bones, which make up the skeleton, are dense, very strong structures and have an ample supply of blood and nerves. Some bones store and manufacture red blood cells in the marrow.

Joints

Joints are held together by ligaments and are found wherever the bones meet. There are two types of joints: movable and immovable. Immovable joints are fused (e.g. the skull). Some movable joints allow slight movement (e.g. vertebrae). Others allow more movement (e.g. ball-and-socket joint of shoulder).

Muscles and tendons

Muscles are mostly (but not all) attached to bones by strong fibrous tissue called tendons. Muscles account for up to 50% of a person's body weight. By contracting and relaxing, muscles move the bones, causing the limbs and digits to move.

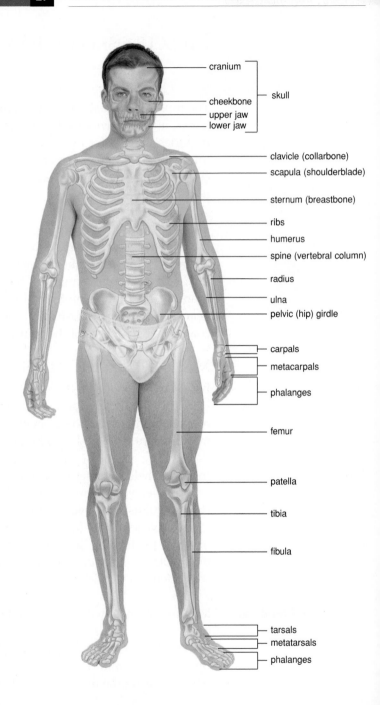

cranium

skull

cheekbone
upper jaw
lower jaw

clavicle (collarbone)
scapula (shoulderblade)

sternum (breastbone)

ribs

humerus

spine (vertebral column)

radius

ulna

pelvic (hip) girdle

carpals
metacarpals

phalanges

femur

patella

tibia

fibula

tarsals
metatarsals
phalanges

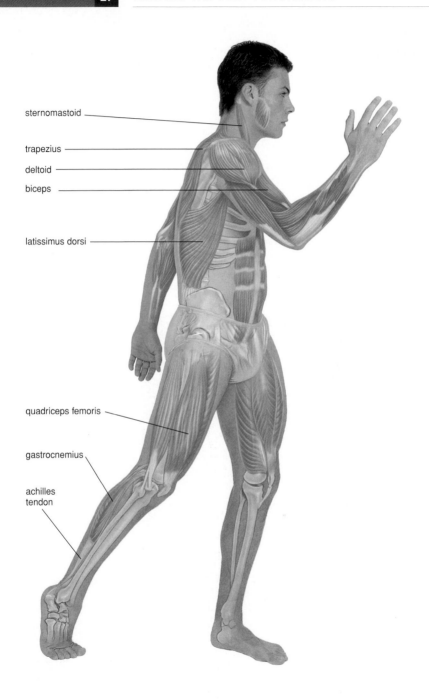

sternomastoid

trapezius

deltoid

biceps

latissimus dorsi

quadriceps femoris

gastrocnemius

achilles
tendon

Glossary

Abdomen part of the body between chest and pelvis, containing digestive organs

Abrasion an open wound caused by direct contact with a rough surface

Acetone a colourless liquid used as a solvent (smells like nail polish remover)

Acid a corrosive substance; a neutraliser of an alkali

Acute pain a pain which is sharp, of sudden onset, severe and short in duration

Afterbirth the placenta, cord and membranes expelled after delivery of baby

AIDS acquired immune deficiency syndrome; condition causing serious illness and death through breakdown in functioning of body's immune system (*see also* HIV)

Airway the passage, starting at mouth or nose, through which air enters and leaves the lungs

Alkali a corrosive substance; a neutraliser of acid

Allergic sensitive to some substance foreign to the body, such as bee venom or certain foods

Alveoli air sacs in the lungs

Amputation cutting off of a limb, digit, or appendage

Anaphylactic shock an extreme and generalised allergic reaction

Angina a heart condition involving acute pain or angina pectoris—unpleasant sensation in chest caused by interference with supply of oxygen to heart, usually brought on by exercise or anxiety

Antiseptic a substance that kills germs or helps to prevent their growth

Anus the external opening of the rectum

Apex pulse heartbeat felt in newborn baby, in chest below left nipple

Artery a vessel through which oxygen-bearing blood is pumped away from the heart

Asphyxia blockage of oxygen supply entering lungs

Aspirate suck out

Assessment evaluation of problems affecting casualty as indicated by history, symptoms and signs observed by first aider

Asthma spasm of bronchial (breathing) tubes in the lungs

Atherosclerosis narrowing of the arteries

Autonomic nervous system the branch of the nervous system that regulates unconscious bodily functions (e.g. sweating)

Avulsion a wound in which skin is partially or completely torn away

Bladder a sac acting as a reservoir, e.g. urinary bladder (for urine), gall bladder (for bile)

Blood pressure the force exerted by blood against walls of blood vessels

Bone marrow soft interior of bones, in which cells are produced

Bowel part of digestive canal below stomach and duodenum

BPC dressing standard British Pharmaceutical Codex dressing

Brachial pulse heartbeat felt on inner upper arm (usually used for infants)

Breastbone flat bone (also called sternum) which forms middle of front of chest and helps separate and support ribs

Bronchi large air passages that divide from windpipe

Capillaries smallest blood vessels

Carbon dioxide a gas which is part of air we breathe out; waste product of human metabolism

Cardiac relating to heart

Cardiopulmonary resuscitation also called CPR— resuscitation technique that combines expired air resuscitation (EAR) with external cardiac compression (ECC)

Carotid pulse heartbeat felt on arteries of neck

Casualty a person, alive or dead, who has suffered an accident or sudden illness

Cells the 'building blocks', microscopic in size, which in their countless millions make up the body

Cerebral relating to brain

Cervical relating to neck

Cholesterol fatty substance which circulates in blood and may be deposited into walls of arteries

Circulation movement of blood through body

Coccyx tail bone—lowest part of spine

Combustible able to be burnt

Communicable diseases caused by germs such as bacteria and viruses, that can be spread from one person to another

Compress a dressing that assists control of bruising and swelling, and helps relieve pain

Concussion any injury to brain, usually caused by a blow, which leads to an altered state of consciousness or to unconsciousness

Constrictive bandage a firmly applied bandage used to control movement of tissue fluid or blood in a limb

Contusion a bruise or closed wound caused by a blow from a blunt object

Convulsions violent and involuntary contractions of limbs and body, accompanied by loss of consciousness (also called seizures or fits)

Corked thigh bruised thigh, with spasm

Cornea clear tissue in front of eye

Corrosive capable of destroying tissue by eating away a surface

CPR cardiopulmonary resuscitation

Cranium skeleton of head, excluding face and jaws

Crater wound caused by tissue being torn from body

Defibrillation application of a controlled electric shock to restore heart rhythm to normal

Dehydration excessive loss of water from body

Diabetes disease caused by loss of insulin-producing cells in pancreas

Diaphragm dome-shaped muscular wall separating abdomen from chest cavity

Diarrhoea overly frequent and soft or liquid bowel motions

Digestive glands the salivary glands, liver, gall bladder and pancreas

Disc a layer of fibro-elastic tissue between the vertebrae

Dislocation injury in which bones of a joint are pushed out of normal contact with each other

Disorientation a state of mental confusion, particularly relating to time and place

Distend swell out, inflate

DRABC stands for Danger, Response, Airway, Breathing, Circulation—the St John universal action plan for first aid management

Dressing material used to cover a wound

Drug any substance, natural or artificial, causing some specific or abnormal physical or mental change

EAR expired air resuscitation

ECC external cardiac compression

Emphysema a chronic condition of the lungs which causes severe restriction of breathing

Envenomation poisoning which results from injection of a venom from bites, stings or penetrating wounds inflicted by reptiles, insects and marine creatures

Epilepsy a condition of the brain leading to seizures or altered conscious states

Expired air resuscitation mouth-to-mouth (or mouth-to-nose and mouth) resuscitation technique used when casualty is unable to breathe; also known as EAR

External cardiac compressions rhythmic compression of heart from outside the body; pressing on breastbone in order to provide artificial circulation of blood; also known as ECC

Extremities fingers and toes

Faeces waste food products passed by the bowel

Fainting a reversible form of loss of consciousness, due to a sudden insufficiency in supply of blood to the brain

Febrile convulsion (*see* Infantile convulsion)

Fibrillation (*see* Ventricular fibrillation)

Flail chest a condition caused by multiple fractures of ribs and instability of rib cage

Floating ribs two pairs of ribs that do not join at the breastbone

Fracture a break in a bone

Gall bladder a sac in upper abdomen which stores bile

Gastroenteritis inflammation of the stomach and intestine, leading to vomiting and/or diarrhoea

Genitals the external reproductive organs

Glands organs that secrete specific substances

Gullet (or oesophagus) the passage from back of throat to stomach

Haematoma an accumulation of blood leaked into tissues from damaged blood vessels resulting from an injury such as a blow

Hallucinations perception of imaginary sights and sounds

Hallucinogen a drug that causes hallucinations

Heart the hollow muscular organ responsible for pumping blood

Heatstroke a serious, life-threatening condition in which body temperature is dangerously high

History when relating to first aid, story of incident or illness, obtained from casualty or witnesses

HIV human immunodeficiency virus—causes clinical illness called AIDS

Hyperextend extend beyond normal position

Hyperglycaemia high blood sugar

Hypertension high blood pressure

Hyperthermia excessive heating of the body

Hyperventilation results from involuntary over-breathing which disturbs oxygen/carbon dioxide balance in the blood

Hypoglycaemia low blood sugar

Hypothermia excessive cooling of the body, usually accidental and often serious

Immobilise to prevent from moving

Incision a cut made by a sharp object

Inebriated drunk

Infantile convulsion caused by rapid rise in temperature in infants and young children (also called febrile convulsion; can also occur in adults)

Infection the invasion and growth of harmful germs in tissues and fluids of body

Inflammation an abnormal state of the tissues characterised by pain, heat, swelling and redness

Insulin a hormone produced in the pancreas which controls level of sugar in blood and body cells

Intestines lower part of alimentary canal

Intoxication a state of excitement, altered conscious state or coma, induced by alcohol or other drugs

Irrigate to wash a wound with a constant stream of water or other fluid

Irukandji a very small stinging jellyfish found in tropical waters of Australia

Jimble small jellyfish most common in coastal waters of South Australia

Laceration a break in skin made by tearing or cutting

Larynx voice box

Lethal deadly

Ligaments tissues connecting or supporting bones at joints

Liver a large organ located in upper abdomen with an important filtering role in digestion; produces bile; metabolises fat etc.

Lungs the pair of breathing organs in the chest cavity

Mallet finger injury to end joint of finger

Medication medicine in any form—liquid, tablet, inhalation or injection

Microorganism a microscopic organism, e.g. germs, virus

Mucus sticky fluid from some parts of body, e.g. nose, bronchi

Nausea a feeling of sickness with possible vomiting

Neonatal newborn or in first four weeks of life

Nerves fibres that convey impulses from one part of body to another

Organ a body part consisting of tissues grouped together to perform a specific function

Oropharyngeal relating to passage that extends from mouth and nasal cavity down to upper end of gullet and windpipe

Oropharyngeal airway a device used to assist in establishing and maintaining an adequate airway

Oropharyngeal aspiration sucking fluid from mouth and nose to prevent inhalation of fluid, and to obtain and maintain an unobstructed airway

Oxygen a life-sustaining gaseous element of air

Pallor paleness of skin

Pancreas a gland that produces insulin and alkaline digestive matter

Paradoxical breathing seen in flail chest injuries—the injured side moves in on inhalation and balloons out on exhalation, instead of, as normal, the other way round

Paralysis inability to move parts of body

Paraplegic paralysed from the waist down

Pelvis the bone structure that forms lowest part of trunk

Perineum pelvic area between genitals and anus

Placenta special tissue attached to mother's uterus, from which unborn baby is nourished and from which umbilical cord emerges

Plasma fluid component of blood

Platelets microscopic cells which float in blood and are involved in the clotting process

Pneumothorax air in chest cavity but outside lung, causing collapse of lung

Post-traumatic occurring after a traumatic experience

Pressure pad firm pad applied over dressing to assist in control of bleeding

Pressure points the points where arteries lie over bones and hence where pressure can be applied to control bleeding

Puffer (or inhaler) device to deliver a regulated dose of asthma medication

Pulmonary relating to lungs

Pulse transmission of heartbeat felt in various parts of the body

Pupil opening in centre of iris (coloured part) of eye

Quadriplegic paralysed from the neck down

Radial pulse heartbeat felt beside crease lines of wrist, on same side as thumb

Rectum final section of alimentary canal ending in the anus

Red cells microscopic discs which float in the plasma of the blood and carry oxygen and carbon dioxide

Respiration breathing

Response a casualty's reply to a first aider's 'shake and shout', enabling assessment of casualty's state of consciousness

Resuscitation reviving a casualty who is unconscious or apparently dead

RICE stands for Rest, Ice, Compression, Elevation—method used by first aiders to manage soft tissue injuries

Sacrum solid bony mass at base of spine which supports pelvis

Scrotum soft pouch hanging from below base of penis, containing the testes

Sedative a drug to calm the nerves

Seizures violent muscular contractions with loss of consciousness (sometimes called fits or convulsions)

Shock a condition in which the circulatory system is not carrying sufficient blood to the tissues

Shoulderblade flat bone of back, jointed with bone of upper arm

Side-effects unintended effects of taking a drug or medicine

Signs features of casualty's condition that can be seen, felt, heard or smelt

Sinus any of the eight cavities in skull that are connected with nasal cavity

Spacer device to improve delivery of asthma medication by a puffer/inhaler

Spasm sudden involuntary muscular contraction

Spinal cord the bundle of nerve tissue extending from base of brain to lower back; surrounded and protected by spine

Spleen an organ in abdomen; helps fight infection

Splint rigid material used to immobilise a limb in treating fractures, dislocations or venomous bites or stings

Sprain stretching of ligaments beyond their normal range

Sputum mucus from lungs, bronchi and throat that is coughed up or spat out through mouth

Sterile free of germs

Sternum breastbone

Stoma artificial opening on body's surface, connecting to a surgically implanted tube (e.g. neck stoma for breathing)

Strain overstretching or overexertion of a muscle

Stroke a condition resulting from a blockage in blood supply to brain, often involving partial paralysis and loss of speech

Suicide taking one's own life

Suffocation death from lack of oxygen

Symptoms what casualty tells you about his or her condition

Testicles the male sex glands located in the scrotum

Tetanus a serious and potentially fatal infection, characterised by muscle spasms

Tissue a group of human body cells that performs a specific function

Toxic poisonous

Trachea windpipe

Trauma a wound, injury or other shocking experience

Triage classification and sorting of casualties for management and evacuation, according to degree of urgency

Umbilical cord the cord attaching unborn baby to placenta in mother's womb

Ureter tube leading from each kidney to bladder

Urine fluid containing waste products removed from blood by kidneys

Vagina passage leading inwards from external female genitalia

Varicose veins swollen veins, usually on the legs

Veins vessels that carry blood towards heart

Venom a toxin (i.e. a poison made by a living thing), usually from a snake, insect, spider or marine creature; secreted and injected by bite or sting

Ventricular fibrillation a chaotic condition of the electrical impulses of the heart, interfering with normal beating

Vertebrae (singular: vertebra) bones that make up spinal column

Vital signs physical signs of life including breathing, heartbeat, consciousness

Voice box (or larynx) part of windpipe where vocal cords are situated

Vomitus stomach contents vomited up

Vulva external female genitals

White cells blood cells which float in plasma and combat infection

Windpipe (or trachea) air tube between throat and lungs

Index

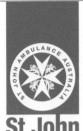

St John

Congratulations
on completing your

You now have immensely valuable skills which will benefit you, your family and your community throughout your life.

Your knowledge of first aid for the injured and distressed will help you make a difference—perhaps the difference between life and death. It's important to keep these skills up-to-date.

The importance of refresher courses and how to book them

- Completing yearly refresher courses offered by St John means your first aid certificate never expires. Maintain your qualification and skills; learn about advances in first aid protocols and practice. In times of crisis, don't rely on fading memory—keep your skill level and certificate up-to-date!

- Book your first aid refresher course by telephoning the St John Ambulance national number. To check when your refresher course is due, look at date of issue on your St John first aid certificate.

Additional first aid training—building on your first aid knowledge

- St John offers many first aid courses at higher levels such as Occupational or Remote Area First Aid. Courses can also be tailored to your particular job, business or lifestyle needs.

To find out more about:

first aid training,

becoming a member of the Operations Branch, or

joining the St John Ambulance Association contact:

Telephone:
Toll free 1300 360 455

Web:
www.stjohn.org.au

E-mail:
training@stjohn.org.au

St John Ambulance first aid course!

Join St John Operations Branch uniformed volunteers

- St John Operations Branch members are highly trained volunteers who, in their familiar black-and-white uniforms, provide vital community support at sporting matches and other public functions.

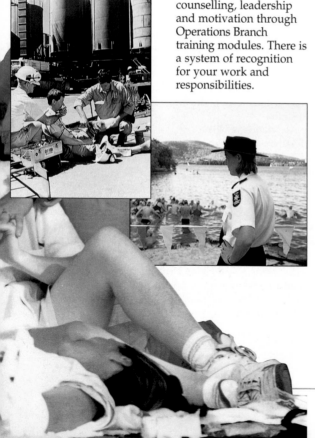

- As a member, you are trained to a highly professional level in first aid including defibrillation, oxygen therapy, burns and exposure, casualty transport and medical emergencies. You will meet other first aiders and share their comradeship and team spirit.

- You can also learn management skills including communication, counselling, leadership and motivation through Operations Branch training modules. There is a system of recognition for your work and responsibilities.

Insurance for first aid certificate holders, through membership in the St John Ambulance Association

- As a newly qualified St John first aider, you may be eligible for membership of the St John Ambulance Association. At a nominal cost per year, everyone who has a current St John Senior (Level 2), Advanced or Occupational First Aid certificate can join.

- All members are covered by a professional indemnity insurance policy which protects against any claims of negligence resulting from rendering first aid as a 'good samaritan'. Insurance does not cover claims arising from first aid given as part of first aiders' paid workplace duties.

Association members receive updates on first aid procedures and other St John news. Be first in line for new first aid products, courses and publications.

ACKNOWLEDGMENTS

St John Ambulance Australia would like to thank all those who have contributed to the development of the *Australian First Aid* project. In particular, the organisation thanks the following groups and individuals for their support:

- St John Ambulance Australia Training Centres
- Members of the St John Ambulance Australia Operations Branch
- Members of the Medical Standards Committee—Professor Paul Gatenby, Dr Bill Griggs, Professor Barry Nurcombe, Professor Michael O'Rourke, Dr Harry Oxer, Associate Professor Fred Leditschke
- Members of the Technical Advisory Committee—Dr Joan Faoagali, Mr Geoff Newman-Martin, Mr Mark Compton, Dr Mark Fitzgerald, Dr Peter Sullivan
- Professor John Pearn, Associate Professor John Williamson, Professor Villis Marshall, Dr Frank Bridgewater, Dr Bernard Stone, Dr Ian Whyte, Associate Professor Jeff Wassertheil, Dr Robert Black, Dr Ray Cook, Mr Robert Luscombe, Mrs Glad Blackstock, Mrs Jill Sterrick, Mr Reg Liddon, Mr Wayne Deakes, Mrs Shirley Dyson, Mr Russell Miller, Ms Rachel Parkinson, Dr Alan Mawdsley, Mr Alan Caust, Mr Mark Pratt (Brighton Life Saving Club), Mr Peter Kyriavou (Sandringham Yacht Club), Mr Kieran Brown
- SANE Australia
- Epilepsy Association of NSW
- National Asthma Campaign
- National Heart Foundation of Australia
- St John Ambulance Canada.

St John Ambulance Australia would also like to thank the following individuals and organisations for supplying photographic material for the book:

- Dr Robert Hartwick, Mr John Lippmann, Mr Douglas Stone, Mr G. Merril
- Flinders University, Royal Flying Doctor Service of Australia, NSW Ambulance Service, Seton Australia Pty Ltd, Kidsafe House Queensland *(see p. 290-291)*, Department of Transport and Regional Development.

Extra illustrations by:
- Ms Erin Knowles.